Advanced Practitioner Handbook

Advanced Practitioner Handbook: Medical Fundamentals

Stevie Park
Queen Elizabeth Hospital Birmingham
UK

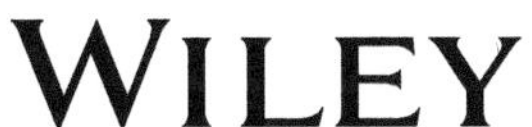

This edition first published 2026

Registered Offices
John Wiley & Sons, Inc., 111 River Street, Hoboken, NJ 07030, USA
John Wiley & Sons Ltd, New Era House, 8 Oldlands Way, Bognor Regis, West Sussex, PO22 9NQ, UK

For details of our global editorial offices, customer services, and more information about Wiley products visit us at www.wiley.com.

The manufacturer's authorized representative according to the EU General Product Safety Regulation is Wiley-VCH GmbH, Boschstr. 12, 69469 Weinheim, Germany, e-mail: Product_Safety@wiley.com.

Wiley also publishes its books in a variety of electronic formats and by print-on-demand. Some content that appears in standard print versions of this book may not be available in other formats.

Library of Congress Cataloging-in-Publication Data Applied for

Paperback ISBN: 9781394303939

Cover Design: Wiley
Cover Image: © miniwide/Shutterstock

Set in 9.5/12.5pt STIXTwoText by Straive, Pondicherry, India

Contents

Preface

Advanced Clinical Practice (ACP) is an essential and evolving part of modern healthcare. It brings together knowledge, skill, and autonomy in a way that bridges the gap between nursing, medicine, and the wider multidisciplinary team (MDT). Yet, despite the importance of the ACP role, I always felt that something was missing – a single, practical, and accessible resource that truly reflected what we do and supported us in learning, studying, and working day-to-day.

That's really where this book began. I wanted to create something for ACPs and those on the journey to becoming one, as well as physician associates, nurses, and other members of the MDT who want to deepen their clinical understanding. My goal was to bring together the kind of information I found myself constantly searching for: clear, detailed explanations grounded in evidence, UK practice, and real-world clinical relevance.

Throughout my own training and experience, I often found that existing texts were too medical, too nursing-focused, or didn't quite capture the unique blend of autonomy and holistic thinking that defines the ACP role. I wanted to bridge that gap – to make something practical, useful, and easy to dip in and out of, whether you're studying for exams, revising a topic, or just looking for clarity on shift.

Each chapter has been written to support that idea: concise but thorough, focused on what really matters in clinical practice. You'll find a balance of pathophysiology, assessment, diagnostics, and management – all tied together with an emphasis on safe, evidence-based, and compassionate care. I hope that it not only informs but also encourages confidence, curiosity, and critical thinking.

Ultimately, this book is for you – for all those striving to grow, to advance their practice, and to keep learning. Whether you're an ACP student, an experienced practitioner, or part of the wider clinical team, I hope these pages become something you can rely on – a reference, a study companion, and maybe even a small source of reassurance on the days when the role feels as challenging as it is rewarding.

April 2026

Stevie Park
West Midlands

Acknowledgements

I would like to extend my heartfelt thanks to everyone who has supported me throughout the creation of this book. First and foremost, to my husband, Kris, who has patiently put up with me, my endless complaining, late-night typing, and occasional mutterings about chapters no one else could understand.

To my son, Callum, you have kept me going, just by being your mom. I am endlessly proud of you.

I am also incredibly grateful to my manager, Rebecca Boot, for her guidance and support throughout this journey, and a special thank you to Team Tate for giving me a space to recharge, sweat out the stress, and pretend that burpees are fun.

Finally, to all of my colleagues, mentors, friends, and family who have inspired, advised, and cheered me on along the way – thank you. This book would not exist without your collective wisdom, patience, and occasional eye rolls.

1

12-Lead ECG Interpretation

The 12-lead electrocardiogram (ECG) is one of the most widely used diagnostic tools in acute and critical care. It provides a rapid, non-invasive assessment of cardiac rhythm, conduction pathways, and evidence of ischaemia, electrolyte disturbances, and structural abnormalities. For advanced practitioners, systematic interpretation is crucial to prevent missed diagnoses and to inform timely management.

A structured approach ensures accuracy and reproducibility. The following framework is widely adopted in UK practice and aligns with the algorithms of the Resuscitation Council UK and guidance from the European Society of Cardiology (ESC).

Step 1: Confirm Patient and Technical Details

Before interpretation, always check that the ECG belongs to the correct patient and that recording standards are met.

- Patient details: full name, date of birth, hospital/NHS number, and date and time of recording.
- Technical settings: confirm paper speed at 25 mm/s and calibration of 10 mm/mV. Incorrect calibration may mimic voltage abnormalities (e.g. low voltage or hypertrophy).
- Artefact: movement, poor electrode contact, or electrical interference may obscure findings.

Step 2: Rate, Rhythm, and Axis

Heart rate: calculate using R–R intervals. At 25 mm/s, 300 divided by the number of large squares between R waves equals the rate in bpm. In irregular rhythms, use a 10 s strip and multiply by 6.

Rhythm

- Is it regular or irregular?
- Is there a P wave before every QRS, and a QRS after every P?
- Assess P-wave morphology (upright in I, II, and aVF; inverted in aVR).

Cardiac axis

- Normal axis: −30° to +90°.
- Left axis deviation: lead I positive, aVF negative. Causes include left anterior fascicular block, LVH, and inferior MI.
- Right axis deviation: lead I negative, aVF positive. Causes include RVH, PE, and lateral MI.
- Extreme axis deviation: lead I negative, aVF negative ('northwest axis') → severe ventricular rhythms.

Step 3: Intervals and Conduction

- PR interval: 120–200 ms (3–5 small squares). Prolonged = first-degree AV block; short = pre-excitation (e.g. WPW).
- QRS duration: ≤120 ms. Wide QRS may indicate bundle branch block, ventricular rhythm, or hyperkalaemia.
- QTc interval: corrected QT <440 ms (men) or <460 ms (women). Prolonged QT intervals increase the risk of torsades de pointes; shortened QT intervals may occur in hypercalcaemia.

Step 4: Regional Lead Groups

Interpretation is improved by grouping leads by anatomical territory and associated coronary arteries.

Region	Leads	Coronary Artery
Inferior	II, III, aVF	Right coronary artery (RCA)
Lateral	I, aVL, V5–V6	Left circumflex (LCx)
Anterior	V1–V4	Left anterior descending (LAD)
Septal	V1–V2	LAD (proximal)

This mapping aids localisation of acute infarction and recognition of reciprocal changes.

Step 5: ST Segment and T-Wave Abnormalities

- ST elevation: hallmark of ST-elevation myocardial infarction (STEMI); must be ≥1 mm in ≥2 contiguous limb leads or ≥2 mm in ≥2 contiguous chest leads. Always correlate with reciprocal depression.
- ST depression: suggests ischaemia, non-ST-elevation myocardial infarction (NSTEMI), or reciprocal changes in STEMI; may also be drug-related (e.g. digoxin effect).

- T-wave inversion: ischaemia, previous MI, PE, or pericarditis.
- Tall, tented T waves: hyperkalaemia.
- Flattened T waves/U waves: hypokalaemia.

Step 6: Common ECG Diagnoses

Diagnosis	Key Features
Atrial fibrillation	Irregularly irregular, absent P waves
Atrial flutter	Sawtooth flutter waves, often 2:1 conduction
Supraventricular tachycardia	Narrow complex, regular, absent P waves
Ventricular tachycardia	Broad QRS, AV dissociation, capture/fusion beats
Heart block	1°, 2° (Mobitz I/II), and 3° complete AV dissociation
STEMI	Localised ST elevation, reciprocal changes
NSTEMI/unstable angina	ST depression, T inversion, raised troponin (NSTEMI)
Electrolyte disorders	Hyperkalaemia: tall T, sine wave; hypokalaemia: U waves

Interpretation Pearls for Advanced Practitioners

- Always compare with previous ECGs to differentiate acute from chronic changes.
- Remember lead aVR: ST elevation here with widespread depression may indicate left main coronary artery occlusion – a high-mortality finding.
- Bundle branch blocks: new left bundle branch block (LBBB) in the context of chest pain may represent STEMI equivalent.
- Be cautious of pacemaker rhythms: they can mask ischaemic changes.
- Artefact, hyperventilation, and hypothermia can mimic pathology.

Bibliography

BMJ Learning. ECG Interpretation Modules. London: BMJ Publishing Group; 2026.

European Society of Cardiology (ESC). Guidelines on acute coronary syndromes. 2023.

National Institute for Health and Care Excellence (NICE). Acute coronary syndromes in adults: NG185. 2024.

RCEMLearning. ECG Library. London: Royal College of Emergency Medicine; 2026.

Resuscitation Council UK. ALS guidelines. 2021.

2

Abdominal Aortic Aneurysm

An abdominal aortic aneurysm (AAA) is defined as a pathological dilatation of the abdominal aorta to a diameter of ≥3.0 cm. Most AAAs occur in the infrarenal segment, just proximal to the aortic bifurcation into the common iliac arteries. Prevalence increases with age and is higher in men, particularly those with cardiovascular risk factors. While many AAAs remain asymptomatic, the natural history involves progressive enlargement, ultimately risking rupture – a catastrophic event with mortality rates of up to 80%.

Risk Factors

Well-recognised risk factors include

- Demographics: male sex, Caucasian ethnicity, and increasing age (>65 years).
- Lifestyle: smoking (the most significant modifiable risk), high alcohol intake, and obesity.
- Medical history: hypertension, hyperlipidaemia, and pre-existing cardiovascular disease.
- Family history: first-degree relatives with AAA carry a higher risk.
- Other associations: connective tissue disorders (e.g. Marfan, Ehlers–Danlos, and Loeys–Dietz), though less common in infrarenal disease.

Pathophysiology

The development of AAA is multifactorial, involving atherosclerotic injury, inflammatory infiltration, and extracellular matrix degradation.

1) Inflammation and oxidative stress
   - Inflammatory cells (neutrophils, macrophages, and T and B lymphocytes) infiltrate the aortic wall.
   - These release proteolytic enzymes and reactive oxygen species, contributing to oxidative stress and tissue injury.
2) Matrix degradation
   - Matrix metalloproteinases (MMPs) degrade elastin and collagen in the tunica media and adventitia.
   - Reduced structural integrity weakens the aortic wall, promoting dilatation.

3) Smooth muscle loss
   - Apoptosis of vascular smooth muscle cells reduces repair capacity.
4) Anatomical location
   - Most AAAs are infrarenal, but they may also be juxta-renal (involving the renal artery origins) or suprarenal.
   - Proximal extension has important implications for surgical planning.

Diagnosis and Screening

Most AAAs are silent until rupture. Proactive detection via screening has transformed outcomes in the United Kingdom.

- National screening programme (NHS AAA screening)
  - All men are invited for an ultrasound scan in the year they turn 65.
  - Women are not routinely screened, though NICE acknowledges that those with a strong family history may benefit.
- Thresholds
  - Normal: <3.0 cm (discharged).
  - Small: 3.0–4.4 cm → annual surveillance.
  - Medium: 4.5–5.4 cm → 3–6 monthly surveillance.
  - Large: ≥5.5 cm → vascular surgery referral within 2 weeks.
- Other diagnostic methods
  - Ultrasound: first-line, non-invasive, and highly sensitive.
    CT angiography (CTA): gold standard for preoperative planning; defines anatomy, involvement of renal/iliac vessels, and presence of thrombus.
  - MRI angiography: an alternative in those intolerant of contrast, though less commonly used.

Management

Management is guided by aneurysm size, rate of expansion, patient comorbidities, and suitability for intervention.

Conservative management (surveillance)

- Suitable for aneurysms <5.5 cm in men or <5.0 cm in women, unless rapid expansion (>1 cm/year).
- Risk factor modification: smoking cessation, blood pressure control, statins, and antiplatelet therapy.
- Regular ultrasound monitoring at intervals dictated by size.

Surgical management

Indicated for:
- Symptomatic aneurysms (pain or tenderness).
- Large aneurysms (≥5.5 cm in men; ≥5.0 cm in women).
- Rapidly expanding aneurysms.

Options

- Open surgical repair (OSR)
  - Involves laparotomy, cross-clamping of the aorta, excision of the aneurysm sac, and insertion of a prosthetic graft.
  - Durable repair with lower long-term complication rates.
  - Higher perioperative morbidity and mortality compared with endovascular aneurysm repair (EVAR).
  - Typically offered to younger, lower-risk patients (<70 years, fit for laparotomy).
- Endovascular aneurysm repair (EVAR)
  - Stent-graft inserted via the femoral arteries under fluoroscopic guidance.
  - Lower perioperative mortality, faster recovery, and shorter hospital stays.
  - Long term: higher re-intervention rates due to endoleaks, graft migration, or occlusion.
  - Fenestrated/branched EVAR (FEVAR/BEVAR): options for complex juxta-renal/suprarenal aneurysms.

The choice of repair depends on anatomical suitability, comorbidity burden, patient preference, and centre expertise.

Ruptured AAA

A ruptured AAA is a surgical emergency with extremely high mortality.

Presentation

- Sudden severe abdominal/back pain.
- Hypotension or shock.
- Pulsatile abdominal mass (classic triad, but not always present).

Immediate management (A–E [airway, breathing, circulation, disability, exposure] approach)

- High-flow oxygen, IV access with bloods (Full Blood Count, Urea & Electrolytes [U&E's] coagulation, crossmatch).
- Permissive hypotension (systolic BP 70–90 mmHg) to maintain organ perfusion without exacerbating bleeding.
- Avoid aggressive fluid resuscitation before haemorrhage control.
- Analgesia and senior involvement.
- Imaging: bedside ultrasound can rapidly confirm diagnosis, but unstable patients should proceed directly to theatre. CTA is preferred if the patient is haemodynamically stable.
- Definitive treatment: urgent OSR or EVAR within 30 minutes of presentation.

Complications

- Endoleak (persistent perfusion of aneurysm sac post-EVAR).
- Graft infection.
- Limb ischaemia due to graft thrombosis.
- Renal impairment from contrast or suprarenal clamping.
- Recurrent aneurysm formation.

Bibliography

BMJ Best Practice. Abdominal Aortic Aneurysm. London: BMJ Publishing Group; 2026.

European Society for Vascular Surgery (ESVS). 2023. *European Society for Vascular Surgery (ESVS) Guidelines on Abdominal Aortic Aneurysm.*

National Institute for Health and Care Excellence (NICE). Abdominal aortic aneurysm: diagnosis and management [NG156]. 2020.

NHS Abdominal Aortic Aneurysm Screening Programme. 2023. *Abdominal Aortic Aneurysm Screening Programme.*

Vascular Society of Great Britain and Ireland. AAA pathway. 2022.

3

Acute Coronary Syndrome

Acute coronary syndrome (ACS) encompasses a spectrum of conditions resulting from myocardial ischaemia due to reduced coronary blood flow. The three main entities are

- ST-elevation myocardial infarction (STEMI)
- Non-ST-elevation myocardial infarction (NSTEMI)
- Unstable angina (UA)

All share a common pathophysiology – rupture or erosion of an atherosclerotic plaque leading to thrombus formation and partial or complete coronary artery occlusion. The clinical severity varies depending on the degree of obstruction, collateral circulation, and duration of ischaemia.

ACS is a leading cause of morbidity and mortality worldwide and represents a true medical emergency. Prompt recognition and treatment are essential to preserve myocardial tissue and improve outcomes.

Clinical Features

Symptoms of ACS are often variable and may be atypical, especially in women, older adults, and individuals with diabetes. Classic features include

- Chest pain: central, heavy, or crushing; radiates to arm, neck, jaw, or back.
- Autonomic symptoms: sweating, nausea, and vomiting.
- Breathlessness: reflects impaired cardiac output or pulmonary oedema.
- Syncope: due to arrhythmia or haemodynamic instability.
- Bradycardia or tachycardia: depending on the ischaemic territory or autonomic response.
- Red flag: silent infarction is more prevalent among diabetic and elderly patients due to autonomic neuropathy.

STEMI

- Defined as new ST-segment elevation in ≥2 contiguous leads (≥1 mm in limb leads, ≥2 mm in chest leads).
- Represents complete coronary artery occlusion → transmural ischaemia.
- Urgent reperfusion is essential (PCI within 120 minutes, or thrombolysis if PCI not available).
- Troponin rise is present but should not delay reperfusion therapy.

NSTEMI

- Presents with ST depression or T-wave inversion on electrocardiogram (ECG), without ST elevation.
- Reflects subtotal occlusion or severe stenosis, allowing some distal flow.
- Diagnosis confirmed by elevated troponin levels, indicating myocardial necrosis.
- Managed with antiplatelets, anticoagulation, and risk stratification for early invasive intervention (PCI).

Unstable Angina

- Like NSTEMI in presentation, but troponin is not elevated.
- Reflects ischaemia without sufficient myocardial injury to release troponin.
- Caused by plaque rupture, thrombus, or vasospasm.
- Requires urgent assessment and anti-ischaemic therapy, as the risk of progression to infarction is high.

Pathophysiology

The primary mechanism in most cases of ACS is the rupture or erosion of an atherosclerotic plaque within a coronary artery. This exposes subendothelial collagen and lipid material to the bloodstream, triggering platelet adhesion, activation, and aggregation. Activated platelets release thromboxane A_2 and adenosine diphosphate (ADP), which enhance platelet recruitment. Simultaneously, the coagulation cascade is activated, generating thrombin and fibrin, which stabilise the platelet plug. The balance between clot formation and endogenous fibrinolysis is disrupted, resulting in a growing thrombus that obstructs blood flow.

The degree of occlusion influences the clinical presentation: a fully occlusive thrombus typically causes transmural ischaemia and an STEMI, whereas partial occlusion results in subendocardial ischaemia, leading to NSTEMI or UA. Additional factors can also contribute, such as dynamic coronary vasospasm (often triggered by cold exposure, cocaine, or stress), distal embolisation of thrombus fragments, and spontaneous coronary artery dissection (SCAD), which is more frequently seen in younger women. The ischaemic cascade begins with impaired relaxation and diastolic dysfunction, followed by systolic wall motion abnormalities, ECG changes, and ultimately chest pain – emphasising the importance of early recognition and intervention.

Investigations

1) ECG
   - First-line, performed within 10 minutes of arrival.
   - Repeat if the initial is non-diagnostic but suspicion remains.
2) Troponin
   - High-sensitivity troponin is the gold-standard biomarker.
   - Rises within 2–4 hours, peaks at 24–48 hours, and can remain elevated up to 14 days.
   - Serial testing at 0 and 3 hours (per NICE NG185).
3) Other investigations
   - Chest X-ray: rule out alternative causes (pneumothorax, aortic dissection, and pneumonia).
   - Echocardiography: assess wall motion abnormalities and complications.
   - Risk stratification: Global Registry of Acute Coronary Events (GRACE) score (predicts mortality and guides invasive strategy).

Initial Management

Core principles are often recalled by the acronym MONA (Morphine, Oxygen, Nitrates, Aspirin), although current practice has evolved.

- Aspirin 300 mg PO immediately.
- Second antiplatelet: ticagrelor or clopidogrel.
- Anticoagulation: Low-molecular-weight-heparin (LMWH) or fondaparinux in NSTEMI/UA.
- Nitrates: sublingual or IV if hypertensive, but avoid in right ventricular infarction.
- Oxygen: only if $SpO_2 < 94\%$.
- Analgesia: IV morphine ± antiemetic.
- Beta-blockers: unless contraindicated (shock, asthma).
- ACE inhibitors and statins: initiated early for secondary prevention.

Reperfusion strategies

- STEMI
  - Primary percutaneous coronary intervention (PCI) (preferred, if available within 120 minutes).
  - Thrombolysis if PCI is not available.

- NSTEMI/UA
  - No immediate thrombolysis.
  - Early invasive strategy (PCI within 24–72 hours) guided by GRACE score.

Complications of ACS

- Arrhythmias: ventricular tachycardia (VT), ventricular fibrillation (VF), brady-arrhythmias, and atrial fibrillation (AF).
- Mechanical complications: papillary muscle rupture → acute MR, ventricular septal rupture, and left ventricular (LV) free wall rupture.
- Cardiogenic shock.
- Pericarditis (Dressler's syndrome).
- Heart failure.

Secondary Prevention

- Dual antiplatelet therapy (DAPT) for 12 months.
- Beta-blockers.
- Angiotensin converting enzyme (ACE) inhibitor/angiotensin II receptor locker (ARB).
- High-intensity statin.
- Lifestyle modification: smoking cessation, diet, and exercise.
- Cardiac rehabilitation.

Bibliography

BMJ Best Practice. Acute Coronary Syndrome. London: BMJ Publishing Group; 2026.

European Society of Cardiology (ESC). Guidelines on acute coronary syndromes. 2023.

National Institute for Health and Care Excellence (NICE). Acute coronary syndromes in adults: diagnosis and management [NG185]. 2020, updated 2024.

Resuscitation Council UK. ALS algorithms. 2021.

4

Acute Kidney Injury

Acute kidney injury (AKI) describes a sudden decline in kidney function, characterised by raised serum creatinine levels and/or reduced urine output. It is a frequent complication in hospitalised patients and is linked with significant morbidity and mortality, particularly in critical care environments. Early detection and prompt management are vital to prevent deterioration and enhance patient outcomes.

Definitions and Criteria

The Kidney Disease: Improving Global Outcomes (KDIGO) criteria are the most widely used and define AKI as the presence of any of the following:

- Increase in serum creatinine by ≥26 µmol/L (≥0.3 mg/dL) within 48 hours.
- Increase in serum creatinine to ≥1.5 times baseline, known or presumed to have occurred within the previous 7 days.
- Urine volume <0.5 mL/kg/h for ≥6 hours.

Staging (KDIGO)

- Stage 1: 1.5–1.9 × baseline creatinine OR ≥26 µmol/L increase; urine output <0.5 mL/kg/h for 6–12 hours.
- Stage 2: 2.0–2.9 × baseline creatinine; urine output <0.5 mL/kg/h for ≥12 hours.
- Stage 3: ≥3.0 × baseline creatinine OR ≥353 µmol/L OR initiation of renal replacement therapy (RRT); urine output <0.3 mL/kg/h for ≥24 hours or anuria for ≥12 hours.

Other classification systems include RIFLE (Risk, Injury, Failure, Loss, ESRD) and AKIN (Acute Kidney Injury Network), although KDIGO integrates and updates both.

Causes of AKI

AKI is typically classified as pre-renal, intrinsic (intra-renal), or post-renal.

Category	Common Causes	Mechanism
Pre-renal	Hypovolaemia (haemorrhage, vomiting, and diarrhoea), sepsis, heart failure, and renal artery stenosis	Reduced renal perfusion

Category	Common Causes	Mechanism
Intrinsic renal	Acute tubular necrosis, glomerulonephritis, interstitial nephritis, vasculitis, and malignant hypertension	Direct injury to renal parenchyma
Post-renal	Prostatic obstruction, ureteric stones, bladder cancer, and retroperitoneal fibrosis	Obstruction to urine flow

Pre-renal causes are the most common and can be potentially reversible if identified early.

Pathophysiology

AKI has a complex and multifactorial pathophysiology, usually triggered by ischaemia, nephrotoxins, or sepsis.

Ischaemic Injury

Reduced renal perfusion causes endothelial dysfunction and severe vasoconstriction, which worsens hypoxia in both the cortex and medulla. The renal medulla is particularly vulnerable due to its high metabolic demand and relatively low oxygen supply.

Cellular Energy Failure

Inadequate perfusion reduces ATP production. ATP depletion impairs ion transport, protein synthesis, and membrane integrity. Failure of Na^+/K^+-ATPase pumps leads to cellular swelling and necrosis.

Oxidative Stress and Inflammation

Hypoxia triggers the production of reactive oxygen species (ROS), which damage lipids, proteins, and DNA. Inflammatory mediators attract immune cells, worsening tissue injury and creating a feedback loop.

Tubular Dysfunction

Nephron function is impaired, with decreased filtration, tubular reabsorption, and secretion. Nephrotoxins can accumulate in the tubular lumen, causing further injury.

Sepsis-Induced AKI

Sepsis adds further complexity, characterised by a systemic inflammatory response, cytokine release, and microvascular dysfunction. Perfusion becomes heterogeneous: some nephrons are hyperperfused while others are hypo-perfused, contributing to patchy injury.

Clinical Features

- Oliguria (<400 mL/day) or anuria.
- Fluid overload (oedema, pulmonary congestion).

- Rising creatinine and urea on blood tests.
- Electrolyte abnormalities (hyperkalaemia, hyponatraemia, and metabolic acidosis).
- Uraemic symptoms in severe cases: confusion, pericarditis, nausea, and bleeding tendency.

AKI often manifests subtly and is identified through routine blood tests before clinical symptoms occur.

Nephrotoxic Drugs

A range of medications can cause or exacerbate AKI.

Drug Class	Examples	Mechanism of Injury
ACE inhibitors/ARBs	Ramipril, losartan	Reduce glomerular filtration pressure by dilating the efferent arteriole
Calcineurin inhibitors	Cyclosporine, tacrolimus	Afferent arteriolar vasoconstriction c→ ↓ GFR
NSAIDs	Ibuprofen, naproxen	Prostaglandin inhibition → afferent vasoconstriction
Aminoglycosides	Gentamicin	Tubular cell toxicity
Amphotericin B, cisplatin	—	Direct tubular toxicity
Rifampin, NSAIDs	—	Interstitial nephritis
Acyclovir, methotrexate	—	Crystal nephropathy → obstruction

A medication history is crucial when assessing AKI.

Management

Management concentrates on early detection, addressing root causes, and providing supportive care.

1) Immediate steps
   - Clinical assessment and observations: BP, fluid balance, and weight.
   - Insert a urinary catheter to monitor output.
   - Bloods: Full blood count (FBC), urea & electrolytes (U&Es), liver function tests (LFTs), coagulation, and cultures if infection suspected.
   - Stop nephrotoxic drugs (NSAIDs, ACEi, and aminoglycosides).
2) Optimise haemodynamics
   - Correct hypovolaemia with IV fluids (balanced crystalloids preferred).
   - Avoid fluid overload – reassess frequently.
   - Treat hypotension with vasopressors if septic shock.

3) Correct biochemical disturbances
   - Hyperkalaemia
     - IV calcium gluconate (cardioprotection).
     - IV insulin with glucose (drives K^+ into cells).
     - Nebulised salbutamol (additional temporary effect).
     - Dialysis if refractory.
   - Metabolic acidosis: may require bicarbonate or dialysis if severe.
4) Relieve obstruction (if post-renal cause)
   - Catheterisation, nephrostomy, or stent, depending on the level of obstruction.
5) Renal Replacement Therapy (RRT) indications include
   - Refractory hyperkalaemia.
   - Severe metabolic acidosis.
   - Pulmonary oedema not responsive to diuretics.
   - Uraemic complications (encephalopathy, pericarditis).

Complications

- Volume overload → pulmonary oedema and hypertension.
- Life-threatening hyperkalaemia.
- Severe metabolic acidosis.
- Uraemia → encephalopathy, pericarditis, and bleeding tendency.
- Progression to chronic kidney disease.

Bibliography

BMJ Best Practice. Acute Kidney Injury. London: BMJ Publishing Group.

KDIGO. KDIGO clinical practice guideline for acute kidney injury. 2021 update.

NICE. Acute kidney injury: prevention, detection and management [NG148]. 2019.

UK Kidney Association. Renal association clinical practice guidelines. 2022.

5

The A–E Assessment

In acute and emergency care, quick recognition and treatment of life-threatening issues are crucial. The A–E (airway, breathing, circulation, disability, exposure) framework offers a systematic assessment method that ensures no vital step is missed. This approach is recommended in Advanced Life Support (ALS), Advanced Trauma Life Support (ATLS), and emergency medicine guidelines throughout the United Kingdom. By prioritising the most immediate threats to life and working from top to bottom, clinicians can provide structured, repeatable care even under intense pressure. Importantly, the A–E assessment is not only an initial survey but also a dynamic process that should be repeated after each intervention, so that improvements or deteriorations are recognised promptly. For advanced practitioners, confidence in applying this structured method is fundamental to safe and effective clinical practice.

Airway

The airway is the top priority in any patient who is acutely unwell or injured because obstruction can lead to hypoxia and death within minutes. Airway compromise can present in various ways, from the noisy stridor caused by upper airway narrowing to gurgling from pooled secretions or complete silence in total obstruction. Clinical vigilance is essential, as reduced consciousness is one of the most common and easily overlooked causes of a threatened airway. Obstruction can be caused by foreign body aspiration, maxillofacial trauma, swelling from anaphylaxis or infection, and depressed airway reflexes due to head injury or overdose.

Initial management concentrates on simple manoeuvres. A head-tilt and chin-lift can relieve soft tissue obstruction in an unconscious patient without cervical spine injury, while a jaw thrust is preferred in trauma to minimise neck movement. Airway adjuncts, such as oropharyngeal or nasopharyngeal airways, may help maintain patency when manual positioning is insufficient. Suction can be used to clear secretions or blood, and high-flow oxygen should be administered early to all critically ill patients.

If these measures are insufficient, escalation to advanced airway interventions becomes necessary. Supraglottic airway devices serve as a temporary solution when intubation is delayed or challenging. Endotracheal intubation remains the gold standard for securing a definitive airway but requires expertise and carries risks, especially in haemodynamically unstable patients. Capnography should always be used to confirm tube placement and monitor ventilation. In rare but catastrophic cases of 'can't intubate, can't oxygenate,' surgical airway access via needle or surgical cricothyroidotomy may be required.

Throughout airway management, clinicians must remember the principle of 'treat as you find': intervene immediately when compromise is recognised rather than waiting until the full A–E assessment is complete. Effective airway management underpins every subsequent stage of evaluation, since no other intervention can succeed without adequate oxygen delivery.

Breathing

Once the airway has been assessed and secured, focus shifts to breathing. The aim at this stage is to determine whether the patient is effectively ventilating and oxygenating. Observation begins with the respiratory rate, a sensitive yet often overlooked indicator of deterioration. A rapid rate may signal distress, sepsis, or metabolic acidosis, while a dangerously low rate can indicate fatigue, opioid toxicity, or neurological depression. Equally important is the breathing pattern and the presence of accessory muscle use, intercostal recession, or paradoxical abdominal movement, all of which suggest significant respiratory compromise. Cyanosis, agitation, or decreased consciousness may also point to inadequate oxygen delivery.

A focused examination should include inspection, palpation, percussion, and auscultation of the chest. Deviation of the trachea, asymmetrical chest movement, or unilateral breath sounds may indicate life-threatening conditions such as tension pneumothorax, while widespread wheeze suggests asthma or COPD exacerbation. Crackles may indicate pulmonary oedema or pneumonia, whereas absent breath sounds over a dull percussion note are consistent with pleural effusion. Oxygen saturation, measured by pulse oximetry, provides rapid information about oxygenation, while arterial blood gases can clarify the presence of hypoxaemia, hypercapnia, or metabolic disturbance.

Initial interventions focus on supporting oxygen delivery. High-concentration oxygen administered via a non-rebreathe mask should be given to critically unwell patients unless there's a clear reason to restrict it, such as in known type 2 respiratory failure where controlled oxygen is preferable. Nebulised bronchodilators, often combined with steroids, can relieve bronchospasm in asthma or COPD. In cases of pulmonary oedema, nitrates and diuretics may be indicated alongside non-invasive ventilation to improve gas exchange.

Where mechanical causes of respiratory failure are identified, prompt intervention is crucial. A tension pneumothorax needs immediate needle decompression followed by chest drain insertion, while large pleural effusions may also require drainage. For severe hypoxaemia unresponsive to standard oxygen therapy, escalation to advanced airway management and mechanical ventilation might be necessary. As with the airway, treatment should be provided as issues are recognised, with reassessment after each intervention to evaluate its effectiveness.

Circulation

After assessing airway and breathing, the next priority is circulation. This stage checks whether the heart and blood vessels are providing enough blood flow to sustain organ function. The first step is a quick clinical assessment, looking for signs of shock such as pallor, sweating, cool extremities, and delayed capillary refill. The pulse is examined for rate, rhythm, and volume; a rapid, weak pulse may indicate hypovolaemia or sepsis, while a slow pulse could suggest conduction issues or drug toxicity. Blood pressure measurement is vital but should be viewed within the overall clinical context, since patients with chronic hypertension may appear stable at 'normal' readings. In contrast, young, healthy individuals can compensate well despite significant hypovolaemia.

Shock can result from several underlying mechanisms. Hypovolaemic shock occurs due to fluid loss, such as haemorrhage or severe dehydration. Cardiogenic shock arises from pump failure, as seen in myocardial infarction or arrhythmias. Distributive shock, most often caused by sepsis, results from vasodilation and increased capillary permeability. Lastly, obstructive shock is caused by physical interference with cardiac filling or output, like tension pneumothorax, cardiac tamponade, or massive pulmonary embolism. Early recognition of the specific type of shock is crucial, as each requires a tailored response.

Management should start by establishing intravenous access, ideally with two large-bore cannulas, and obtaining initial blood tests, including a full blood count, renal profile, and clotting studies. Additionally, group and save or crossmatch should be performed if bleeding is suspected. A cardiac monitor should be attached to assess rhythm and identify arrhythmias, while an ECG can detect acute coronary syndromes or conduction abnormalities. Intravenous fluids are essential for initial resuscitation in hypovolaemic or distributive shock, but caution is necessary to avoid fluid overload, especially in cardiogenic shock. Vasopressors, such as noradrenaline, may be required to improve perfusion if fluids are insufficient, particularly in cases of septic shock.

In cases of life-threatening arrhythmia, immediate intervention may be necessary. Ventricular fibrillation or pulseless ventricular tachycardia requires prompt defibrillation, while bradyarrhythmias might respond to atropine, external pacing, or temporary pacing wires. External haemorrhage should be controlled with direct pressure, tourniquets, or haemostatic dressings, whereas internal bleeding often needs surgical or interventional radiology assistance. Circulatory support is a dynamic process that involves constant reassessment of pulse, blood pressure, urine output, and lactate levels to guide ongoing treatment.

Disability

Once circulation has been stabilised, the patient's neurological status should be assessed. This stage, summarised as 'Disability', involves a quick but structured assessment of consciousness, pupils, and blood glucose, as changes in these can indicate primary neurological issues or secondary effects of systemic illness. The level of consciousness is most often evaluated using the AVPU scale (Alert, Responds to Voice, Responds to Pain, Unresponsive) for a rapid bedside impression, or the more detailed Glasgow Coma Scale (GCS), which provides a consistent score based on eye, verbal, and motor responses. A decreasing GCS is a key red flag that calls for urgent investigation and potential intervention to safeguard the airway.

Examination of the pupils provides additional information about neurological function. Unequal or poorly reactive pupils may indicate raised intracranial pressure, cranial nerve injury, or intracranial haemorrhage. Additionally, assessment of limb strength and movement can reveal lateralising neurological deficits suggestive of stroke or seizure activity. At this stage, it is essential to check blood glucose, as hypoglycaemia is a reversible cause of reduced consciousness and seizures that can easily mimic more serious neurological conditions.

Management during the disability assessment concentrates on correcting reversible problems. Hypoglycaemia should be treated promptly with intravenous glucose, and seizures controlled with benzodiazepines. Patients with markedly reduced consciousness or recurrent seizures may need airway protection and escalation to intensive care. Rapid recognition of stroke syndromes is crucial to initiate reperfusion therapies where suitable, while signs of raised intracranial pressure require urgent neurosurgical input. Disability should always be considered in the broader clinical context to identify and treat reversible causes before irreversible damage occurs.

Exposure

The final stage of the structured assessment is Exposure, which involves a complete head-to-toe examination of the patient. This requires fully uncovering the patient to look for hidden injuries, rashes, surgical scars, bleeding, or signs of infection such as cellulitis. It also includes examining pressure areas and lines or drains for complications. While doing this, it is essential to preserve the patient's dignity and comfort, keeping them covered where possible and ensuring a warm environment. Hypothermia is common in critically ill patients and contributes to coagulopathy, acidosis, and worsening shock, so active warming with blankets, warmed IV fluids, or specialised devices may be required.

Exposure also enables clinicians to synthesise findings from earlier parts of the assessment. For instance, an abdominal examination may uncover rigidity or distension, which can account for hypotension, or limb swelling may indicate a source of sepsis. In trauma, systematic exposure assists in identifying bleeding sources that might have been overlooked during the primary survey. Throughout this stage, the practitioner should bear in mind that exposure is not a one-off event but an ongoing process, with reassessment as new information arises.

Reassessment and Summary

The A–E framework is not meant as a one-off checklist, but as a continuous cycle. After each intervention, the assessment should be repeated to review the response and identify any deterioration. For example, after intubation, reassessing breathing ensures sufficient ventilation, while after fluid resuscitation, circulation should be checked to confirm improved perfusion. Reassessment promotes safety and helps prioritise in dynamic situations where multiple issues may occur simultaneously.

In summary, the A–E assessment offers a clear and reproducible framework for managing patients who are acutely unwell. By working methodically from airway to exposure and addressing life-threatening issues as they arise, practitioners lower the chance of missing diagnoses and improve outcomes. For advanced practitioners, mastering this approach supports safe clinical decision-making and leadership during emergencies. Its significance is not only in the initial assessment but also in its flexibility, as repeating the cycle allows for the recognition and prompt treatment of evolving problems. The A–E assessment is thus the foundation of emergency care, combining clinical skill with a structured set of priorities to protect patient survival.

Bibliography

American College of Surgeons Committee on Trauma. Advanced Trauma Life Support (ATLS) Student Course Manual. 10th ed. Chicago: ACS; 2018.

BMJ Best Practice. Initial Assessment of The Acutely Ill Patient. BMJ Publishing Group; 2023.

Inada-Kim M et al. The National Early Warning Score 2 (NEWS2) in acute care: standardising the assessment of illness severity in the NHS. Clin Med (Lond). 2019;19(3):203–207.

National Institute for Health and Care Excellence (NICE). Acutely Ill Adults in Hospital: Recognising and Responding to Deterioration (CG50). London: NICE; 2007, updated 2019.

Resuscitation Council UK. Advanced Life Support (ALS) Guidelines. London: RCUK; 2021.

Royal College of Emergency Medicine (RCEM). Emergency Department Clinical Guidelines. London: RCEM; 2022.

Thim T, Krarup NH, Grove EL, Rohde CV, Løfgren B. Initial assessment and treatment with the Airway, Breathing, Circulation, Disability, Exposure (ABCDE) approach. Int J Gen Med. 2012;5:117–121.

6

Addison's Disease

Addison's disease is the most common form of adrenal insufficiency, caused by either adrenal cortex damage or decreased hormone production. It is categorised as primary hypoadrenalism associated with autoimmune disease.

It leads to insufficient production of cortisol, aldosterone, and adrenal androgens. Cortisol deficiency disrupts metabolism, immune response, and stress adaptation, while aldosterone deficiency causes electrolyte imbalance and dehydration. Dysfunction in the hypothalamic–pituitary–adrenal axis leads to elevated corticotropin-releasing hormone and adrenocorticotropic hormone (ACTH).

Pathophysiology

A deficiency of cortisol disrupts multiple homeostatic mechanisms. It is a vital regulator of glucose metabolism by stimulating gluconeogenesis. When this process fails, it can cause hypoglycaemia. Its absence also reduces the negative feedback on the hypothalamic–pituitary axis, leading to increased levels of ACTH. Cortisol also has anti-inflammatory and immunosuppressive effects, which can be impaired, worsening an autoimmune response and heightening susceptibility to infections.

Aldosterone deficiency causes impaired renal sodium reabsorption and potassium excretion, leading to hyponatraemia, hyperkalaemia, and hypovolaemic hypotension. The decreased volume prompts a compensatory rise in renin; however, without enough aldosterone, this process will eventually fail, resulting in further hypotension. This imbalance can also lead to metabolic acidosis due to disturbed hydrogen ion regulation.

Presentation

- Hyperpigmentation of the skin
- Hypoglycaemia
- Hypotension
- GI disturbances
- Weight loss or anorexia
- Fatigue and muscle weakness

Treatment

Hydrocortisone is typically used in acute situations, such as an adrenal crisis, for glucocorticoid replacement because of its short duration of action and similarity to the body's natural cortisol production.

A longer-acting glucocorticoid, prednisolone, is typically used to maintain a steady concentration for long-term management.

Fludrocortisone is usually used for mineralocorticoid replacement to supplement the aldosterone typically produced by the adrenal glands.

Steroids should never be stopped suddenly.

Useful Blood Tests

Cortisol: Monitoring cortisol levels can assist in diagnosing Addison's disease or other medical conditions or help determine whether a prescribed steroid dose is too high or too low.

ACTH stimulation test: This assesses how well the adrenal glands work. ACTH is the hormone that stimulates the adrenal glands to produce cortisol.

Other Investigations

Sodium levels may decrease, while potassium and calcium levels could rise due to low mineralocorticoid levels.

Glucose levels may be low, particularly in children.

Adrenal antibodies will confirm the cause of adrenal insufficiency once a diagnosis is established.

A CT scan to assess the adrenal glands and identify any calcification.

Bibliography

BMJ Best Practice. Addison's Disease. London: BMJ Publishing Group.

Bornstein SR et al. Diagnosis and treatment of primary adrenal insufficiency: an endocrine society clinical practice guideline. J Clin Endocrinol Metab. 2016;101(2):364–389.

NICE. Adrenal insufficiency: diagnosis and management. NG524, 2023.

Society for Endocrinology UK. Adrenal crisis guidelines. 2020.

7

Advanced Life Support (ALS)

Advanced Life Support (ALS) builds on Basic Life Support (BLS), offering advanced interventions for patients in cardiac arrest or peri-arrest conditions. ALS focuses on early recognition, rapid initiation of effective chest compressions, early defibrillation in shockable rhythms, sophisticated airway management, drug therapy, and addressing reversible causes. In the UK, ALS training and protocols are guided by the Resuscitation Council UK (RCUK) and are regularly revised to align with the European Resuscitation Council (ERC) guidelines.

ALS is designed not only for managing cardiac arrest but also for the structured treatment of peri-arrest arrhythmias such as severe bradycardia or tachycardia, aiming to prevent progression to cardiac arrest.

Basic Principles

Key principles of ALS include

1) Early recognition and prevention
   - Identify deteriorating patients early using tools like NEWS2.
   - Call for help (2222/medical emergency team).
2) High-quality chest compressions
   - Depth 5–6 cm, rate 100–120/min, allow full chest recoil.
   - Minimise interruptions (<10 seconds).
3) Defibrillation
   - Immediate defibrillation for shockable rhythms (ventricular fibrillation [VF]/pulseless ventricular tachycardia [pVT]).
   - Use biphasic waveform defibrillators (150–200 J).
4) Airway and breathing
   - Bag–mask ventilation initially.
   - Advanced airway (supraglottic device, intubation) by trained providers.
   - 100% oxygen during resuscitation.
5) Circulation and drugs
   - Establish IV/IO access.
   - Adrenaline and amiodarone are the main pharmacological agents in cardiac arrest.
6) Reversible causes (4 Hs and 4 Ts)
   - Must always be sought and corrected during resuscitation.

Reversible Causes (4 Hs and 4 Ts)

Cause	Key Features	Treatment
Hypoxia	Low SpO_2, cyanosis, airway obstruction	Airway manoeuvres, oxygen, and intubation if needed
Hypovolaemia	History of bleeding, trauma, and shock	IV/IO fluids, blood products
Hypothermia	Core temp <35°C	Active/passive rewarming
Hyper/ hypokalaemia, metabolic disorders	ECG changes, metabolic acidosis	HyperK^+: IV calcium, insulin + glucose, salbutamol, dialysis. HypoK^+: IV potassium
Tension pneumothorax	Unilateral absent breath sounds, distended chest	Immediate needle decompression, chest drain
Tamponade	Raised jugular venous pressure muffled heart sounds, and hypotension	Pericardiocentesis
Toxins	Drug overdose, poisoning	Antidotes, supportive care
Thrombosis (coronary or pulmonary)	Acute coronary syndrome (ACS), massive PE	percutaneous coronary intervention (PCI) for myocardial nfarction (MI), thrombolysis/ embolectomy for pulmonary embolism (PE)

Cardiac Arrest Algorithm

Shockable rhythms

- Ventricular fibrillation (VF)
- Pulseless ventricular tachycardia (pVT)

Algorithm

1) Confirm arrest → call for help.
2) Start CPR (30:2). Attach defibrillator/monitor.
3) If VF/pVT: defibrillate immediately (150–200 J biphasic).
4) Resume CPR immediately for 2 minutes.
5) Reassess rhythm → shock again if VF/pVT persists.
6) Adrenaline 1 mg IV/IO after the third shock, then every 3–5 minutes.
7) Amiodarone 300 mg IV after the third shock; additional 150 mg after fifth shock if needed.
8) Continue CPR, rhythm checks every 2 minutes, correct reversible causes.

Non-shockable rhythms

- Asystole
- Pulseless electrical activity (PEA)

Algorithm

1) Confirm arrest → call for help.
2) Start CPR immediately.
3) Adrenaline 1 mg IV/IO ASAP, then every 3–5 minutes.
4) Continue CPR for 2 minutes, rhythm check.
5) If organised rhythm returns, check for pulse → return of spontaneous circulation (ROSC) care.
6) Continue until reversible causes are corrected or resuscitation is deemed futile.

Peri-Arrest Rhythms

Bradycardia (see ALS bradycardia algorithm)

- Atropine 500 mcg IV; repeat every 3–5 minutes (max 3 mg).
- If ineffective: transcutaneous pacing, IV isoprenaline/adrenaline infusion, and transvenous pacing if available.

Tachycardia with a pulse (see ALS tachycardia algorithm)

- Broad complex: assume ventricular tachycardia (VT) until proven otherwise → amiodarone; cardioversion if unstable.
- Narrow complex: vagal manoeuvres, adenosine, and beta-blockers if persistent.

Post-Resuscitation Care

Survival from cardiac arrest depends not only on the ROSC but also on post-resuscitation care.

- ABCDE assessment.
- Maintain SpO_2 94–98%; avoid hyperoxia.
- Targeted temperature management (TTM) for comatose patients.
- 12-lead electrocardiogram (ECG): consider emergency PCI if STEMI.
- Blood pressure support: IV fluids and vasopressors.
- Treat underlying cause (infection, MI, PE, electrolyte disorders).
- Admit to critical care for monitoring and ongoing care.

Cardioversion

Cardioversion is used to restore sinus rhythm in tachyarrhythmias and can be either electrical (synchronised DC shock) or pharmacological (antiarrhythmic drugs).

Indications (unstable rhythms → urgent DC shock)

- Atrial fibrillation/flutter with haemodynamic instability.
- Supra ventricular tachycardia (SVT) resistant to vagal manoeuvres/adenosine.
- Monomorphic VT with a pulse.

Key points for electrical cardioversion

- Synchronise shock with R wave (avoid R-on-T).
- Energy settings (biphasic): AF 120–200 J; VT 100 J; flutter/SVT 50–100 J.
- Sedation required if elective.
- Contraindications: atrial thrombus, digoxin toxicity, and electrolyte disturbances.

Pharmacological options (elective or stable patients)

- Flecainide (if no structural heart disease).
- Amiodarone (if LV dysfunction/structural disease).
- Beta-blockers, diltiazem, or verapamil for rate control if rhythm control is not appropriate.

Bibliography

European Resuscitation Council (ERC). Guidelines for resuscitation. 2021.

Guidelines. Resuscitation council UK ALS tachycardia algorithm; NICE NG196 (AF); ESC AF guidelines. 2020.

Resuscitation Council UK. Adult advanced life support guidelines. 2021.

Soar J et al. Adult advanced life support guidelines and supporting publication. Resuscitation. 2021;161:115–151.

8

Airway Assessment and Intubation

Securing the airway is a core aspect of critical care and emergency medicine. Effective management requires rapid recognition of airway compromise, a systematic assessment to foresee potential difficulties, and preparation for definitive airway interventions.

Airway Assessment

A systematic approach helps in forecasting and handling potential challenges.

- LEMON mnemonic
  - Look externally (facial trauma, obesity, and large tongue).
  - Evaluate 3-3-2 rule (mouth opening >3 fingers, hyoid-chin >3 fingers, thyroid-floor >2 fingers).
  - Mallampati score (visualisation of oropharyngeal structures).
  - Obstruction (tumour, abscess, and stridor).
  - Neck mobility (cervical collar and arthritis).

Signs of impending airway compromise include stridor, hypoxia despite oxygen therapy, altered consciousness, and rapidly progressing swelling of the face and neck.

Preparation

Safe intubation relies on thorough preparation.

- SOAP ME: suction, oxygen (bag–valve mask or high-flow), airway equipment (endotracheal tube [ETT] bougie, and supraglottic device), pharmacology (sedative and paralytic), monitoring (SpO_2, ECG, and BP), and end-tidal CO_2.
- Pre-oxygenation: 3–5 minutes of 100% oxygen reduces desaturation risk.
- Drugs: rapid sequence induction (RSI) involves an induction agent (e.g. propofol, ketamine, and etomidate) and a paralytic (suxamethonium or rocuronium). Choice depends on haemodynamics and contraindications.

Intubation Procedure

- Positioning: sniffing position or ramped for obese patients.
- Laryngoscopy: direct (Macintosh) or video laryngoscope.
- Tube placement: endotracheal tube (size 7.0–8.0 mm adults) passed through the vocal cords.
- Confirmation: the gold standard is waveform capnography. Supportive signs include bilateral chest rise, equal breath sounds, absence of gastric sounds, and a chest X-ray (CXR) confirming the tube tip 2–5 cm above the carina.

Post-Intubation Care

- Secure the tube and commence appropriate sedation/analgesia.
- Initiate mechanical ventilation tailored to the condition (e.g. lung-protective strategy in acute respiratory distress syndrome [ARDS]).
- Continuous monitoring: SpO_2, $EtCO_2$, and haemodynamics.

Complications

- Immediate: hypoxia, hypotension, aspiration, and oesophageal intubation.
- Delayed: ventilator-associated pneumonia, barotrauma, and laryngeal injury.
- Failed intubation: insert a supraglottic device or follow the difficult airway algorithm. If 'can't intubate, can't oxygenate' (CICO), perform front-of-neck access (cricothyroidotomy).

Bibliography

Apfelbaum JL et al. Practice guidelines for management of the difficult airway: an updated report by the ASA task force on difficult airway management. Anesthesiology. 2022;136(1):31–81.

Difficult Airway Society (DAS). DAS guidelines for the management of the unanticipated difficult intubation in adults. 2020.

Royal College of Anaesthetists. Airway management – curriculum resources. 2022.

9

Anaemia

Anaemia is characterised by a reduction in the blood's ability to carry oxygen, primarily caused by a decrease in red blood cell (RBC) mass, haemoglobin levels, or haematocrit. It is a syndrome rather than a single disease, with multiple underlying causes that need to be identified for proper treatment.

According to the WHO, anaemia affects over 1.6 billion people worldwide, making it a significant public health concern. It is particularly common among women of childbearing age, children, and individuals with chronic illnesses. Clinically, anaemia manifests as fatigue, pallor, dyspnoea, or reduced organ perfusion, but its severity and symptoms can vary depending on the underlying cause and the rate at which it develops.

Normal ranges

- Women: 115–165 g/L
- Men: 130–180 g/L

Classification by mean corpuscular volume (MCV)

Mean corpuscular volume (MCV) provides a useful framework for the initial classification of anaemia.

- Microcytic anaemia: MCV <80 fL
- Normocytic anaemia: MCV 80–100 fL
- Macrocytic anaemia: MCV >100 fL

Microcytic Anaemia

Microcytic anaemia occurs due to impaired haemoglobin synthesis, which causes increased mitotic divisions of RBC precursors, resulting in smaller, paler cells (hypochromia).

Causes

- Iron deficiency anaemia (IDA): most common worldwide; secondary to chronic blood loss (menorrhagia and GI bleeding), poor diet, malabsorption (e.g. coeliac disease), or increased demand (pregnancy).
- Thalassaemia: inherited defect in globin chain synthesis.

- Sideroblastic anaemia: failure of iron incorporation into haem due to congenital enzyme defects, toxins (lead, alcohol), or drugs (isoniazid).
- Anaemia of chronic disease: sometimes presents microcytically due to hepcidin-mediated iron sequestration.

Clinical features

- General: fatigue, pallor, and exertional dyspnoea.
- Specific to IDA: brittle nails, koilonychia (spoon nails), angular stomatitis, and pica.

Investigations

- FBC: low Hb, low mean cell volume (MCV), and low mean corpuscular haemoglobin (MCH).
- Iron studies: ↓ ferritin, ↓ serum iron, and ↑ total iron-binding capacity (TIBC) (in IDA).
- Hb electrophoresis (for thalassaemia).
- Bone marrow (rarely needed).

Management

- Treat underlying cause (exclude GI malignancy in older adults).
- Oral iron (ferrous sulphate/fumarate) for 3–6 months after Hb normalises.
- IV iron if malabsorption, intolerance, or severe deficiency.
- Blood transfusion for severe symptomatic anaemia.

Normocytic Anaemia

MCV remains normal, but overall RBC counts are reduced due to decreased production or increased destruction.

Causes

- Anaemia of chronic disease: inflammatory cytokines induce hepcidin, trapping iron in storage and suppressing erythropoiesis.
- Haemolysis: autoimmune haemolytic anaemia (AIHA), hereditary spherocytosis, glucose-6-phosphate dehydrogenase (G6PD) deficiency, and sickle cell disease.
- Bone marrow failure: aplastic anaemia and marrow infiltration (leukaemia, myeloma, and lymphoma).
- Acute blood loss.

Clinical features

- Fatigue, pallor, and exertional dyspnoea.
- Haemolysis-specific: jaundice, dark urine, and splenomegaly.
- Bone marrow infiltration: bone pain and pancytopenia signs.

Investigations

- Reticulocyte count (↑ in haemolysis and ↓ in marrow failure).
- Haemolysis screen: LDH ↑, indirect bilirubin ↑, haptoglobin ↓, and Coombs test (autoimmune).
- U&Es to check renal function.
- Bone marrow biopsy if marrow infiltration is suspected.

Management

- Treat underlying cause (control inflammation, immunosuppression for AIHA, and chemotherapy for malignancy).
- Erythropoiesis-stimulating agents (ESAs) in chronic kidney disease (CKD).
- Transfusion in severe cases.

Macrocytic Anaemia

Macrocytosis occurs when DNA synthesis is impaired, resulting in delayed nuclear maturation while the cytoplasm enlarges.

Causes

- Megaloblastic: vitamin B12 deficiency (pernicious anaemia, malabsorption, gastrectomy, and vegan diet) and folate deficiency (diet, alcohol, and methotrexate).
- Non-megaloblastic: alcohol excess, liver disease, hypothyroidism, reticulocytosis, and myelodysplastic syndromes.

Clinical features

- General anaemia symptoms.
- B12 deficiency: glossitis, neuropathy, peripheral paraesthesia, and subacute combined degeneration of the spinal cord.
- Folate deficiency: glossitis, but no neurological signs.

Investigations

- FBC: high MCV, hyper-segmented neutrophils on blood film (megaloblastic).
- Serum B12 and folate.
- Homocysteine ↑ in both; methylmalonic acid ↑ only in B12 deficiency.
- Liver function tests and thyroid function tests if non-megaloblastic suspected.

Management

- B12 deficiency: IM hydroxocobalamin lifelong (pernicious anaemia) or until the cause is corrected.
- Folate deficiency: oral folic acid (after ruling out B12 deficiency to avoid worsening neurological complications).
- Address alcohol use and treat underlying liver or thyroid disease.

Clinical Summary Table

Anaemia Type	Causes	Key Tests	Key Features	Management
Microcytic	IDA, thalassaemia, sideroblastic, and anaemia of chronic disease (ACD)	FBC, ferritin, and iron studies	Fatigue, pallor, and koilonychia	Iron and treat cause
Normocytic	ACD, haemolysis, bone marrow failure, and acute blood loss	Reticulocyte count and haemolysis screen	Jaundice and splenomegaly	Treat cause, ESA, and transfusion
Macrocytic	B12/folate deficiency, alcohol, liver disease, and hypothyroid	B12, folate, homocysteine, and methylmalonic acid (MMA)	Glossitis and neuro signs (B12)	B12 injections and folate

Bibliography

BMJ Best Practice. Anaemia. London: BMJ Publishing Group; 2026.

British Society for Haematology. Guidelines for the diagnosis and management of iron deficiency anaemia. 2021.

Hoffbrand AV, Moss PA. Essential Haematology. 8th ed. Wiley-Blackwell; 2019.

NICE. Anaemia – iron deficiency. NG130, 2019.

10

Anaphylaxis

Anaphylaxis is a severe, life-threatening allergic reaction that occurs in sensitised individuals after exposure to a specific allergen. The severity depends on the type of allergen, route of exposure, amount, and individual sensitivity.

Pathophysiology

Anaphylaxis is an acute, systemic hypersensitivity reaction primarily caused by immunoglobulin E (IgE). During the initial exposure to an allergen, sensitisation occurs with the production of allergen-specific IgE antibodies. These IgE antibodies bind to high-affinity receptors (FcεRI) on the surface of mast cells and basophils, effectively 'arming' them for future exposure.

Upon re-exposure to the same allergen, cross linking of the bound IgE antibodies on these sensitised mast cells and basophils induces rapid degranulation. This process releases pre-formed and newly synthesised inflammatory mediators, including

- Histamine: causes vasodilation, increases vascular permeability (resulting in fluid leakage and swelling), induces smooth muscle contraction in airways, and stimulates nerve endings, leading to itching.
- Leukotrienes and prostaglandins: enhance bronchoconstriction, raise vascular permeability, and promote mucus secretion.
- Cytokines and chemokines: attract more immune cells, boosting the inflammatory response.

The widespread vasodilation caused by this leads to a quick drop in systemic vascular resistance and hypotension. Increased vascular permeability results in plasma leaking into interstitial tissues, contributing to angioedema and hypovolaemia. Smooth muscle contraction causes bronchospasm and laryngeal oedema, which can severely compromise the airway. These combined effects reduce tissue perfusion and oxygen delivery, risking shock and multi-organ failure.

Additionally, the release of systemic mediators directly affects the heart by increasing heart rate and myocardial contractility as a compensatory response. However, coronary vasoconstriction and decreased perfusion may lead to arrhythmias or cardiac arrest.

Non-IgE-mediated anaphylactoid reactions cause similar symptoms through direct mast cell activation without prior sensitisation. Triggers include specific medications (e.g. NSAIDs and opioids), contrast agents, and physical stimuli such as exercise.

Risk Factors

- Atopy raises the risk of death during anaphylaxis but does not raise its occurrence.
- Higher risk in patients with asthma or on beta-blockers/angiotensin converting enzyme inhibitors.

Management of Anaphylaxis

Step	Action	Notes
Initial ABC approach	Secure airway, obtain IV access, and give 100% oxygen	Lower the head of the bed to improve venous return
Remove cause	Identify and eliminate allergen exposure	
Adrenaline	0.5 mg IM (0.5 mL of 1:1000 solution) every 5 minutes as needed	Monitor BP, pulse, and respiratory function; continue until BP recovers
If no response to adrenaline	Prepare for rapid intubation	Reduces the need for cricothyroidotomy
Adrenaline caution	IV adrenaline dose is much lower than IM dose	Avoid overdose
Antihistamines	Chlorphenamine 10 mg IV	Adjunctive treatment, not a substitute for adrenaline
Corticosteroids	Hydrocortisone 200 mg IV	Helps prevent biphasic reactions
Fluid resuscitation	IV saline to treat hypotension	Monitor blood pressure
Treat bronchospasm	Inhaled β2-agonists	For asthmatic wheeze

Bibliography

British Society for Allergy and Clinical Immunology. BSACI Guideline for the Diagnosis and Management of Anaphylaxis. London: BSACI; 2021 https://www.bsaci.org.

Davidson's Principles and Practice of Medicine. 24th ed. Edinburgh: Elsevier; 2022.

Kumar and Clark's Clinical Medicine. 11th ed. Edinburgh: Elsevier; 2023.

McLean, Tooke SJ, Bethune A, Fay F, Spickett RA. Adrenaline in the treatment of anaphylaxis: What is the evidence? BMJ. 2003;327(7427):1332–1335.

National Institute for Health and Care Excellence. Anaphylaxis: Assessment and Referral after Emergency Treatment (CG134). London: NICE; 2020 https://www.nice.org.uk.

NHS. Anaphylaxis; 2023. https://www.nhs.uk

Oxford Handbook of Clinical Medicine. 11th ed. Oxford: Oxford University Press; 2024.

Resuscitation Council UK. Emergency Treatment of Anaphylaxis: Guidelines for Healthcare Providers. London: Resuscitation Council UK; 2021 https://www.resus.org.uk.

Ring J, Worm M, Kim JSH. Anaphylaxis. Nat. Rev. Disease Primers. 2014;1:1–20.

World Allergy Organization. *World Allergy Organization anaphylaxis guidance 2020*. World Allergy Organization J. 2020;13(10):1–25.

11

Antibiotics

Antibiotics are among the most significant discoveries in modern medicine. They are essential for managing sepsis, pneumonia, meningitis, and many other bacterial infections. Antibiotics also support surgical procedures, transplantation, and cancer chemotherapy by lowering the risk of infectious complications.

However, the advantages of antibiotics are threatened by the rise of antimicrobial resistance (AMR). Inappropriate prescribing, overuse in both healthcare and agriculture, and global inequalities in access have all contributed to resistance becoming a major public health crisis. The World Health Organisation (WHO) recognises AMR as one of the top ten global health threats, and antibiotic stewardship has become a fundamental part of medical practice.

Mechanisms of Action

Antibiotics work by targeting bacterial structures or processes that are absent in human cells, ensuring selective toxicity. The main mechanisms are

1) Inhibition of cell wall synthesis
   - The bacterial cell wall consists of peptidoglycan, which offers structural strength.
   - Drugs such as beta-lactams (penicillins, cephalosporins, carbapenems, monobactams) and glycopeptides (vancomycin, teicoplanin) disrupt peptidoglycan cross linking, causing bacterial lysis.
   - Beta-lactams bind to penicillin-binding proteins (PBPs), whereas glycopeptides bind directly to cell wall precursors.
   - These drugs are bactericidal and primarily effective against Gram-positive organisms, although some also have activity against Gram-negative bacteria.
2) Disruption of cell membranes
   - Some antibiotics disrupt membrane integrity, leading to leakage of cellular contents.
   - Examples include polymyxins (e.g. colistin), which target Gram-negative bacteria, and daptomycin, which acts against Gram-positive organisms.
   - These agents are often reserved for multidrug-resistant infections due to toxicity concerns.

3) Inhibition of protein synthesis
   - Bacterial ribosomes (70S) differ from human ribosomes (80S), offering a selective target.
   - Antibiotics can bind to the 30S or 50S ribosomal subunit to inhibit translation.
   - Key classes include
     - Aminoglycosides (gentamicin, amikacin) – cause misreading of mRNA; bactericidal.
     - Macrolides (erythromycin, clarithromycin, azithromycin) – prevent translocation; bacteriostatic.
     - Tetracyclines (doxycycline, minocycline) – block tRNA binding; broad-spectrum.
     - Clindamycin – inhibits peptide bond formation, effective in anaerobic infections.
4) Inhibition of nucleic acid synthesis
   - Fluoroquinolones (ciprofloxacin, levofloxacin) inhibit DNA gyrase and topoisomerase IV, thereby preventing DNA replication.
   - Rifamycins (rifampicin) inhibit RNA polymerase and are used in treating tuberculosis and prosthetic joint infections.
   - Metronidazole damages DNA through free radical formation and is highly effective against anaerobes and protozoa.
5) Antimetabolite activity
   - Antibiotics can disrupt vital metabolic pathways.
   - Sulphonamides and trimethoprim inhibit folate synthesis, which bacteria need for DNA replication.
   - When used together (co-trimoxazole), they exhibit synergistic bactericidal activity.

Major Antibiotic Classes

Beta-Lactams

Beta-lactam antibiotics are the most frequently used group of antibacterials. They contain a standard beta-lactam ring and work by inhibiting bacterial cell wall synthesis. Resistance often develops through beta-lactamase enzymes, alterations in PBPs, or reduced drug permeability.

Penicillins

- Benzylpenicillin (penicillin G): very effective against *Streptococcus pyogenes* and *Treponema pallidum*. Its use is limited by widespread resistance.
- Flucloxacillin: essential medication for *Staphylococcus aureus* infections (excluding methicllin-resistant *Staphylococcus aureus* [MRSA]).
- Amoxicillin/ampicillin: provides wider Gram-positive and some Gram-negative coverage; commonly used in respiratory and urinary tract infections.
- Co-amoxiclav: combines amoxicillin with clavulanic acid, a beta-lactamase inhibitor, broadening its spectrum against resistant organisms.

Cephalosporins

Divided into 'generations' with escalating Gram-negative activity.

- 1st generation (cefazolin, cephalexin): covers Gram-positive bacteria, used for skin and soft tissue infections.
- 2nd generation (cefuroxime): broader Gram-negative coverage, used in pneumonia.
- 3rd generation (ceftriaxone, ceftazidime): offers excellent Gram-negative coverage and crosses the blood–brain barrier (used in meningitis).
- 4th generation (cefepime): broader Gram-negative and *Pseudomonas* activity.
- 5th generation (ceftaroline): effective against MRSA.

Carbapenems (e.g. Meropenem, Imipenem)

- Extremely broad-spectrum, covering Gram-positives, Gram-negatives (including *Pseudomonas*), and anaerobes.
- Considered 'last-resort' agents; resistance (e.g. carbapenemase-producing Enterobacterales) is a primary global concern.

Monobactams

- Aztreonam provides Gram-negative coverage, including *Pseudomonas*. It is often used for patients allergic to penicillin.

Glycopeptides (e.g. Vancomycin, Teicoplanin)

- Inhibit cell wall synthesis at a site different from beta-lactams.
- Effective solely against Gram-positive organisms, including MRSA and enterococci.
- Therapeutic drug monitoring is required because of nephrotoxicity.

Aminoglycosides (e.g. Gentamicin, Amikacin)

- Inhibit protein synthesis via the 30S ribosomal subunit.
- Potent, bactericidal drugs that kill in a concentration-dependent manner.
- Effective against aerobic Gram-negative bacilli; utilised in sepsis and synergistic with beta-lactams for endocarditis.
- Toxicities: nephrotoxicity and ototoxicity → dosing requires careful monitoring.

Macrolides (e.g. Erythromycin, Clarithromycin, Azithromycin)

- Inhibit protein synthesis through the 50S ribosomal subunit.
- Effective against Gram-positive cocci and atypical organisms (e.g. *Mycoplasma pneumoniae*, *Chlamydia*, *Legionella*).
- Commonly used for respiratory tract infections and as a penicillin alternative in cases of allergy.
- Adverse effects: gastrointestinal upset, QT prolongation, and CYP450 interactions.

Tetracyclines (e.g. Doxycycline, Minocycline, Tigecycline)

- Broad-spectrum, effective against Gram-positive, Gram-negative, and atypical pathogens.
- Uses include treating acne, respiratory tract infections, and zoonoses (e.g. Lyme disease, rickettsial infections).
- Contraindicated in children under 12 years and pregnant women due to effects on teeth and bones.
- Resistance is becoming more widespread.

Fluoroquinolones (e.g. Ciprofloxacin, Levofloxacin, Moxifloxacin)

- Inhibit DNA gyrase and topoisomerase IV.
- Excellent Gram-negative activity, including *Pseudomonas* (ciprofloxacin).
- Levofloxacin and moxifloxacin provide respiratory coverage.
- Side effects include tendon rupture, QT prolongation, and CNS effects – leading to restrictions on routine prescribing (Medicines and Healthcare products Regulatory Agency [MHRA] guidance).

Sulphonamides and Trimethoprim

- Inhibit folate synthesis; used alone (trimethoprim in UTIs) or in combination (co-trimoxazole) for *Pneumocystis jirovecii* pneumonia and resistant Gram-negative bacteria.
- Growing resistance restricts the use of trimethoprim as empirical therapy in many regions.

Oxazolidinones (e.g. Linezolid)

- Effective against Gram-positive organisms, including MRSA and vancomycin-resistant enterococci (VRE).
- Excellent oral bioavailability, making them useful in step-down therapy.
- Adverse effects: myelosuppression and neuropathy with prolonged use.

Other Important Agents

- Metronidazole: effective against anaerobes and protozoa; commonly used in intra-abdominal infections and *Clostridioides difficile* colitis.
- Daptomycin: rapidly bactericidal against Gram-positives; utilised in resistant endocarditis and bloodstream infections (not for pneumonia).
- Chloramphenicol: broad-spectrum but restricted by bone marrow suppression; still employed in meningitis within low-resource settings.

Antibiotic Stewardship

Antibiotic stewardship involves coordinated strategies aimed at optimising antimicrobial use, improving patient outcomes, and decreasing resistance. It is a fundamental duty for all clinicians.

Principles of Stewardship

1) Right drug, right dose, right duration, and right route.
2) Use the narrowest effective spectrum to minimise collateral damage.
3) De-escalate therapy once culture results are available.
4) Avoid antibiotics for viral infections or asymptomatic bacteriuria, except during pregnancy or prior to urological procedures.
5) Review ongoing prescriptions daily – many infections need shorter courses than commonly used.

Strategies in Practice

- Guideline adherence: NICE and local trust protocols should guide empiric therapy.
- IV-to-oral switch: many antibiotics have excellent oral bioavailability (e.g. linezolid, ciprofloxacin, doxycycline), allowing early step-down from IV therapy.
- Antibiotic 'time-outs': reassess therapy at 48–72 hours once cultures return.
- Restriction policies: reserve critical drugs (e.g. carbapenems, colistin) for proven resistant infections.

Benefits of Stewardship

- Reduces AMR.
- Minimises risk of *C. difficile* infection.
- Improves patient safety by reducing drug toxicity.
- Conserves healthcare resources by shortening hospital stays and reducing unnecessary prescribing.

Bibliography

European Centre for Disease Prevention and Control (ECDC). Antimicrobial Resistance Surveillance in Europe 2022. Stockholm: ECDC; 2023.

Bennett JE, Dolin R, Blaser MJ, eds. Mandell, Douglas, and Bennett's Principles and Practice of Infectious Diseases. 9th ed. Philadelphia: Elsevier; 2020.

National Institute for Health and Care Excellence (NICE). Antimicrobial Stewardship: Systems and Processes for Effective Antimicrobial Medicine Use. NICE Guideline [NG15]. London: NICE; 2015, updated 2023.

O'Neill J. Tackling Drug-Resistant Infections Globally: Final Report and Recommendations. The Review on Antimicrobial Resistance. London: HM Government/Wellcome Trust; 2016.

Piddock LJV. The crisis of no new antibiotics—what is the way forward? Lancet Infect Dis. 2012;12(3):249–253.

Public Health England. Start Smart – Then Focus: Antimicrobial Stewardship Toolkit for English Hospitals. London: PHE; 2015.

The British National Formulary (BNF). Antibacterials. London: BMJ Group and Pharmaceutical Press; 2020.

The Sanford Guide to Antimicrobial Therapy. 50th Edition. Sperryville, VA: Antimicrobial Therapy, Inc.; 2020.

World Health Organization (WHO). Global Action Plan on Antimicrobial Resistance. Geneva: WHO; 2015.

12

Acute Respiratory Distress Syndrome (ARDS)

Definition

Acute respiratory distress syndrome (ARDS) is a severe, diffuse inflammatory injury of the lungs that causes increased pulmonary vascular permeability, decreased aerated lung tissue, and hypoxaemia. Bilateral radiographic opacities, decreased compliance, increased lung weight, and impaired gas exchange characterise it.

The 2024 updated definition permits diagnosis in both intubated and non-intubated patients.

Diagnostic Criteria

ARDS is diagnosed when the following criteria are met:

- Acute onset (within 1 week of a known insult).
- Bilateral opacities on chest X-ray, CT, or ultrasound (not explained by effusions, collapse, or nodules).
- Hypoxaemia
  - PaO_2/FiO_2 ratio ≤ 300 mmHg (≤40.0 kPa) or
  - SpO_2/FiO_2 ratio ≤ 315 mmHg (≤42.0 kPa).

Severity is classified by oxygenation impairment:

- Mild: PaO_2/FiO_2 200–300 mmHg (26.7–40.0 kPa).
- Moderate: 100–200 mmHg (13.3–26.7 kPa).
- Severe: ≤100 mmHg (≤13.3 kPa).

Pathophysiology

ARDS results from either direct lung injury, such as pneumonia or aspiration, or from indirect systemic insults, including sepsis, trauma, or pancreatitis. Regardless of the trigger, the subsequent pathological processes share standard features that disrupt alveolar-capillary integrity, impair gas exchange, and decrease lung compliance. The condition progresses through distinct, though sometimes overlapping, phases.

Exudative Phase (First 7 Days)

The initial stage involves damage to the alveolar-capillary barrier. This injury allows protein-rich oedema to flood into the alveoli, overwhelming normal clearance mechanisms. Inflammatory cells, especially neutrophils, infiltrate the lung tissue and release cytokines, proteases, and reactive oxygen species. These mediators worsen tissue damage and contribute to the formation of hyaline membranes, which further hinder oxygen exchange.

Proliferative Phase (7–14 Days)

During the proliferative phase, type II pneumocytes and fibroblasts multiply to restore the epithelial lining and repair tissue damage. However, inflammation often continues, and in some patients, this phase signals the beginning of early fibrotic changes. The alveolar structure becomes progressively more abnormal, with impaired surfactant production and reduced elasticity.

Fibrotic Phase (After 14 Days in Some Patients)

In some patients, ARDS advances to a fibrotic stage. Excessive collagen accumulation and scarring replace healthy lung tissue, resulting in a significant decrease in lung compliance and diffusion capacity. This chronic scarring severely limits gas exchange and results in prolonged dependence on ventilators and poor functional recovery.

Resolution

Resolution of ARDS is achievable, although the progression varies considerably. Over time, alveolar fluid is reabsorbed, and some epithelial cells undergo repair. However, many patients are left with residual abnormalities, such as restrictive lung disease or decreased exercise tolerance, indicating incomplete lung recovery.

Additional Mechanisms

Several additional mechanisms contribute to the pathophysiology of ARDS. Surfactant dysfunction promotes alveolar collapse, worsening ventilation–perfusion (V/Q) mismatch, and refractory hypoxaemia results from severe mismatch and shunt physiology. Meanwhile, pulmonary hypertension may develop due to vascular injury, microthrombosis, and vasoconstriction, adding further stress to right ventricular function.

Management

There is no curative treatment; care remains supportive, with an emphasis on improving oxygenation and minimising ventilator-induced injury.

- Protective lung ventilation
  - Tidal volume 6 mL/kg predicted body weight.
  - Plateau pressure < 30 cmH_2O.
  - Accept permissive hypercapnia.
- Prone positioning
  - ≥16 hours/day in moderate–severe ARDS.
  - Improves oxygenation and survival.
- Positive end expiratory pressure(PEEP) and recruitment manoeuvres
  - Use PEEP to maintain alveolar recruitment.
  - Recruitment manoeuvres (30–40 cm H_2O for 30 seconds) can be considered in refractory hypoxaemia.
- Adjuncts
  - Inhaled nitric oxide (iNO) may improve V/Q mismatch transiently.
  - Conservative fluid management once shock is stabilised.
- Steroids
  - Current evidence does not support routine steroid use in ARDS.
- Rescue therapies
  - Veno-venous extracorporeal membrane oxygenation in refractory hypoxaemia despite optimal ventilation.

Bibliography

ARDS Definition Task Force. Update on ARDS diagnostic criteria. JAMA. 2024:342.

ARDSNet. Ventilation with lower tidal volumes as compared with traditional tidal volumes for ARDS. N Engl J Med. 2000;342(18):1301–1308.

Fan E et al. An official ATS/ESICM/SCCM clinical practice guideline: mechanical ventilation in ARDS. Am J Respir Crit Care Med. 2017.

NICE. NICE clinical knowledge summary: acute respiratory distress syndrome. 2023.

13

Arterial Blood Gas (ABG)

An arterial blood gas (ABG) is a key bedside test used to evaluate oxygenation, ventilation, and acid–base status. Blood is usually taken from the radial artery (preferred due to its easy access and collateral circulation), the femoral artery, or through an arterial line in critically ill patients. Since the procedure can be painful, a local anaesthetic should be administered to alert patients.

Acid–Base Balance

The body maintains pH within a narrow range of 7.35–7.45, which is crucial for enzyme activity, cardiac rhythm stability, and efficient oxygen delivery. Even minor deviations can impair cellular function.

Acid–base homeostasis is regulated by

1) Buffers (especially the bicarbonate buffer system).
2) Lungs (rapid CO_2 regulation).
3) Kidneys (slower regulation of H^+ and HCO_3^-).

A change in pH is described as

- Acidosis: $pH < 7.35$.
- Alkalosis: $pH > 7.45$.

The Bicarbonate Buffer System

The key buffer is the carbonic acid–bicarbonate system:

$$CO_2 + H_2O \rightleftharpoons H_2CO_3 \rightleftharpoons H^+ + HCO_3^- \; CO_2 + H_2O \rightleftharpoons H_2CO_3 \rightleftharpoons H^+ + HCO_3^- \; CO_2 + H_2O \rightleftharpoons H_2CO_3 \rightleftharpoons H^+ + HCO_3^-$$

- The lungs regulate CO_2 (an acid) by altering ventilation.
- The kidneys regulate HCO_3^- and H^+, reabsorbing or excreting to maintain long-term balance.

Compensation

- In acidosis (↑H^+) → kidneys reabsorb HCO_3^- and excrete H^+.
- In alkalosis (↓H^+) → kidneys excrete HCO_3^- and retain H^+.
- Respiratory changes occur rapidly (minutes to hours).
- Metabolic compensation is slower (hours to days).

Normal ABG Values

Parameter	Normal Range	Notes
pH	7.35–7.45	Acid–base balance
PaO_2	10–13 kPa	Oxygenation
$PaCO_2$	4–7 kPa	Ventilation
HCO_3^-	22 – 26 mmol/L	Metabolic component
Base excess	−2 to +2 mmol/L	Indicates metabolic contribution

Interpretation Framework

A structured approach ensures errors are avoided:

1) Check pH – acidosis or alkalosis?
2) Assess $PaCO_2$ – is it respiratory?
3) Assess HCO_3^-/base excess – is it metabolic?
4) Decide if compensation is present
   - Respiratory versus metabolic cause.
   - Fully, partially, or uncompensated.
5) Assess oxygenation (PaO_2/FiO_2 ratio) – to detect hypoxaemia.

Key Patterns

Disorder	pH	$PaCO_2$	HCO_3^-	Notes
Respiratory acidosis	↓ (<7.35)	↑ (>6.0)	Normal/↑	Hypoventilation, COPD, and CNS depression
Respiratory alkalosis	↑ (>7.45)	↓ (<4.5)	Normal/↓	hyperventilation, anxiety, and sepsis
Metabolic acidosis	↓	Normal/↓	↓ (<22)	Shock, renal failure, diabetic keto-acidosis (DKA), and sepsis
Metabolic Alkalosis	↑	Normal/↑	↑ (>26)	Vomiting, diuretics, and hypokalaemia

Clinical Relevance

- Hypoxaemia ($PaO_2 < 8\,kPa$): suggests impaired oxygenation → pneumonia, acute respiratory distress syndrome (ARDS), and pulmonary embolism.
- Hypercapnia ($PaCO_2 > 6.5\,kPa$): suggests hypoventilation → COPD exacerbation, neuromuscular weakness, and CNS depression.
- Lactate: frequently measured alongside ABG; elevated in shock, sepsis, and tissue hypoperfusion.

Bibliography

Gattinoni L et al. Understanding blood gases in the ICU. Intensive Care Med. 2021:44.
NICE Clinical Knowledge Summary. Acid–base disorders. 2023.
Resuscitation Council UK. Peri-arrest ABG interpretation guidelines. 2022.

14

Asthma

Asthma is a chronic inflammatory disorder of the airways characterised by variable and reversible airway obstruction, bronchial hyperresponsiveness, and persistent inflammation. It presents with episodic symptoms such as wheezing, dyspnoea, chest tightness, and cough, particularly at night or in the early morning. It is one of the most common long-term respiratory conditions worldwide and remains a leading cause of morbidity despite advances in treatment.

Pathophysiology

Asthma results from a complex interaction of genetic factors, environmental triggers, and an immune system imbalance. The primary abnormality is airway inflammation, which causes bronchial hyperresponsiveness and airflow obstruction.

When exposed to allergens or irritants, immune cells – particularly mast cells, eosinophils, and T-lymphocytes – become activated. These cells release a cascade of inflammatory mediators, including histamine, leukotrienes, and prostaglandins. These mediators cause the following:

- Bronchoconstriction (via airway smooth muscle contraction).
- Mucosal oedema, increasing airway resistance.
- Mucus hypersecretion further narrows the lumen.

Over time, persistent inflammation can cause airway remodelling, where structural changes reduce reversibility and worsen disease progression. These include smooth muscle hypertrophy, goblet cell hyperplasia, and subepithelial fibrosis.

Diagnosis

Asthma is primarily a clinical diagnosis, confirmed by objective evidence of fluctuating airflow obstruction.

- Peak expiratory flow (PEF): diurnal variation >20%.
- Spirometry: obstructive pattern (↓Forced expiratory volume (FEV_1), ↓FEV_1/Forced vital capacity (FVC) ratio); reversibility post-bronchodilator with FEV_1 improvement ≥12% and ≥200 mL.

- Fractional exhaled nitric oxide (FeNO): elevated in eosinophilic inflammation.
- Allergy testing: skin prick or serum-specific IgE may identify triggers.

Classification of Severity

Asthma severity is evaluated based on symptom burden, nocturnal awakenings, use of reliever medication, activity limitations, and spirometry results.

Severity	Features
Intermittent	<2 days/week symptoms and <2 night-time symptoms/month
Mild	>2 days/week, minor limitation, and FEV_1 ≥80% predicted
Moderate	Daily symptoms, some limitation, and FEV_1 60–80% predicted
Severe	Symptoms throughout the day, frequent night-time symptoms, and FEV_1 <60% predicted

Red Flags – Life-Threatening Features

- Silent chest, cyanosis, or exhaustion.
- SpO_2 <92% or a normal/raised $PaCO_2$ (suggesting impending respiratory failure).
- Bradycardia, hypotension, or altered consciousness.
- Inability to complete sentences or Peak expiratory flow rate (PEFR) <33% predicted.

Acute Management

Stage	Action and Details
Initial Assessment	Use the A–E approach. Assess airway, RR, SpO_2, accessory muscle use, consciousness, and speech. Record HR, BP, and temperature. Check PEFR against predicted or personal best. Blood gases in severe cases (look for rising CO_2/acidosis). Auscultate for wheeze, silent chest (life-threatening), or added sounds.
Oxygen Therapy	High-flow O_2, target saturations 94–98% (or 88–92% in CO_2 retainers).
First-Line Medications	• Nebulised/inhaled salbutamol (short-acting beta antagonist [SABA]): 2.5–5 mg every 20 minutes initially, oxygen-driven. • Ipratropium bromide (short-acting muscaranic antagonist [SAMA]): 500 mcg every 4–6 hours, often combined with salbutamol in severe/life-threatening asthma. • Systemic corticosteroids: oral prednisolone 40–50 mg for 5–7 days, or IV hydrocortisone 100 mg if unable to take orally.
Monitoring and Escalation	Reassess response: PEFR, RR, HR, SpO_2. Consider continuous nebulisation if requiring SABA more often than every 2 hours. Escalate early if no improvement.

Stage	Action and Details
Adjunct Therapies	• IV magnesium sulphate 1.2–2 g over 20 mins for severe/life-threatening asthma. • IV aminophylline in critical care if refractory to inhaled therapy (loading 5 mg/kg, then infusion). • IV ketamine may be used in refractory status asthmaticus (1 mg/kg bolus, then infusion).
Antibiotics	Only if evidence of bacterial infection.
Ventilatory Support	Consider Continuous Positive Airway Pressure (CPAP) / Bilevel Positive Airway Pressure (BPAP) in deteriorating patients. Intubation and invasive ventilation may be required in respiratory arrest, exhaustion, or refractory hypoxaemia/hypercapnia – but carries high risk due to dynamic hyperinflation and barotrauma.

Long-Term Management

- Inhaled corticosteroids (ICS) remain the cornerstone for persistent asthma.
- Step-up therapy includes long-acting beta antagonists (LABA's), leukotriene receptor antagonists, or biologics (omalizumab, mepolizumab) for severe eosinophilic asthma.
- Patient education, trigger avoidance, and personalised asthma action plans are essential for long-term control.:

Bibliography

BTS/SIGN. British guideline on the management of asthma. 2023 update.

Global Initiative for Asthma (GINA) Report. 2024.

Levy ML, Beasley R, Bostock B, et al. A simple and effective evidence-based approach to asthma management: ICS-formoterol reliever therapy. Br. J. General Practice. 2024;74:86–89.

NICE NG245. Asthma: diagnosis, monitoring and chronic asthma management. 2024.

15

Blood and Blood Products

Red Blood Cells (RBCs)

Red blood cells (RBCs) are concentrated erythrocytes with most plasma removed, supplying the oxygen-carrying element of blood.

Indications

- Symptomatic anaemia causing tissue hypoxia.
- Acute blood loss where volume replacement is insufficient.
- Chronic anaemia unresponsive to other treatment.

Mechanism

Transfused RBCs primarily restore oxygen delivery through haemoglobin, a tetrameric protein with four heme groups that reversibly bind oxygen. Increasing circulating RBC mass enhances tissue oxygenation and supports cellular metabolism. RBC transfusion also aids in maintaining blood viscosity, promoting microvascular perfusion.

Platelets

Platelet concentrates are either pooled or obtained through apheresis and suspended in plasma.

Indications

- Prophylaxis and treatment of bleeding in thrombocytopenia ($<10\text{–}20 \times 10^9$/L).
- Platelet dysfunction or consumption coagulopathies.
- Pre-procedure prophylaxis in thrombocytopenic patients.

Mechanism

Platelets maintain haemostasis through

1) Adhesion to exposed collagen via GPIb and von Willebrand factor.
2) Activation with shape change and mediator release (ADP, thromboxane A_2).
3) Aggregation via GPIIb/IIIa-fibrinogen cross linking.
4) Surface provision for coagulation factor assembly, amplifying thrombin and fibrin generation.

Fresh Frozen Plasma (FFP)

Fresh frozen plasma (FFP) is the plasma component of blood, frozen soon after donation, containing all coagulation factors.

Indications

- Active bleeding with coagulopathy.
- Emergency reversal of warfarin.
- Liver disease–associated coagulopathy.
- Massive transfusion protocols.

Mechanism

FFP replenishes clotting factors (fibrinogen, prothrombin, factors V, VII, VIII, IX, X, XI, XII, XIII) and natural anticoagulants (antithrombin, protein C/S). This restores haemostatic balance and supplies limited amounts of albumin and immunoglobulins, aiding in maintaining osmotic pressure and immune defence.

Cryoprecipitate

Cryoprecipitate is a cold-insoluble plasma fraction rich in fibrinogen, factor VIII, von Willebrand factor, and factor XIII.

Indications

- Hypofibrinogenaemia (fibrinogen < 1.5 g/L).
- Massive transfusion with ongoing bleeding.
- Disseminated intravascular coagulation (DIC).
- Certain clotting factor deficiencies.

Mechanism

Cryoprecipitate supplies concentrated fibrinogen for forming the fibrin mesh, factor VIII for the intrinsic pathway, von Willebrand factor for platelet adhesion, and factor XIII for cross-linking fibrin. Collectively, these support stable clot formation and adequate haemostasis.

Bibliography

Estcourt LJ et al. Guidelines for the use of platelet transfusions. Br J Haematol. 2017;176.

Levy JH, Goodnough LT. How I use fibrinogen replacement therapy in acquired bleeding. Blood. 2015;125.

NHS Blood and Transplant (NHSBT). Handbook of Transfusion Medicine. 6th ed; 2023.

NICE NG24. Blood Transfusion. 2022.

16

Blood Film

A blood film (peripheral blood smear) is a simple but vital diagnostic tool used to assess the morphology of red blood cells (RBCs), white blood cells (WBCs), and platelets. While the full blood count (FBC) provides quantitative data, the blood film offers essential qualitative information, often guiding diagnosis in haematology and general medicine.

Erythrocytes

Normal erythrocytes are biconcave discs, 6–8 μm in diameter, with central pallor occupying one-third of the cell. Deviations from this morphology may indicate underlying pathology.

- Microcytosis: small RBCs, often due to iron deficiency anaemia or thalassaemia.
- Macrocytosis: large RBCs, associated with vitamin B12/folate deficiency, alcohol use, or myelodysplastic syndromes.
- Hypochromia: increased central pallor from reduced haemoglobin content.
- Target cells: bullseye appearance, seen in liver disease and thalassaemia.
- Spherocytes: round, dense cells without central pallor, associated with hereditary spherocytosis or autoimmune haemolysis.
- Schistocytes: irregularly shaped fragments, suggestive of microangiopathic haemolysis (e.g. disseminated intravascular coagulation [DIC], thrombotic thrombocytopenic purpura [TTP], hemolytic uremic syndrome [HUS]).
- Sickle cells: crescent-shaped cells typical of sickle cell disease.

Leukocytes

White cell morphology offers insight into infection, inflammation, or haematological malignancy.

- Neutrophilia: often due to bacterial infection, steroids, or stress.
- Toxic granulation/vacuolation: seen in severe sepsis.

- Atypical lymphocytes: large, irregular cells common in viral infections (e.g. Epstein Barr virus [EBV]).
- Blast cells: immature cells suggestive of acute leukaemia – urgent further investigation required.
- Hypersegmented neutrophils: typically found in megaloblastic anaemia (B12/folate deficiency).
- Eosinophilia: may indicate allergy, parasitic infection, or hypereosinophilic syndromes.

Platelets

Platelet assessment is helpful for both quantitative and qualitative disorders:

- Thrombocytopenia: low numbers may be immune-mediated, drug-induced, or marrow-related.
- Large platelets: suggest increased platelet turnover (e.g. immune thrombocytopenia).
- Platelet clumping: can lead to spuriously low automated counts (pseudothrombocytopenia).

Clinical Utility

A blood film remains a highly valuable diagnostic tool in a wide range of clinical settings. It is often requested when investigating cases of unexplained anaemia, helping to differentiate between various underlying causes such as nutritional deficiencies, bone marrow failure, or haemolysis. It is equally important in the assessment of pancytopenia or isolated cytopenias, as it can offer clues as to whether the issue originates in the bone marrow or results from peripheral destruction. When haemolysis is suspected, the presence of fragmented RBCs on a blood film provides a quick and direct way to confirm the diagnosis. Blood films also play a central role in diagnosing and classifying haematological malignancies, such as leukaemia, lymphoma, and myeloma, as they allow examination of abnormal or immature cells. Beyond diagnosis, they remain an essential tool for monitoring response to therapy, whether assessing recovery after chemotherapy or evaluating the effectiveness of vitamin replacements in cases of deficiency. This makes the blood film not only a diagnostic cornerstone but also a helpful guide in ongoing patient management.

Bibliography

Bain BJ. Blood Cells: A Practical Guide. 5th ed. Wiley-Blackwell; 2015.

Hoffbrand AV, Moss PAH. Essential Haematology. 8th ed. Wiley-Blackwell; 2019.

NICE NG24. Blood Transfusion. 2022.

17

Bowel Obstruction

Bowel obstruction refers to a mechanical or functional blockage of the intestines that prevents the normal passage of bowel contents. It can occur in the small intestine (small bowel obstruction, SBO) or the large intestine (large bowel obstruction, LBO). Alternatively, disruption of coordinated peristalsis without a physical blockage is known as functional obstruction (ileus). Prompt recognition and treatment are vital, as untreated obstruction can lead to ischaemia, perforation, and sepsis.

Causes of Bowel Obstruction

Small Bowel Obstruction (SBO)	Large Bowel Obstruction (LBO)	Functional Causes (Ileus)
Adhesions (post-operative)	Colorectal carcinoma	Post-operative ileus
Hernias (inguinal, femoral)	Volvulus (sigmoid, caecal)	Electrolyte disturbances (e.g. hypokalaemia)
Intussusception	Diverticulitis with stricture	Medications (opioids, anticholinergics)
Crohn's disease strictures	Faecal impaction	Severe systemic illness or sepsis
Gallstone ileus	Inflammatory strictures (inflammatory bowel disease)	Neurological disease (e.g. Parkinson's disease)
Tumours or foreign bodies	Ischaemic colitis strictures	Endocrine/metabolic (e.g. hypothyroidism)

Clinical Features

Symptom	Description
Abdominal pain	Colicky in mechanical SBO; constant, severe in strangulation
Vomiting	Early in SBO; feculent in distal obstruction
Abdominal distension	Prominent in LBO
Constipation/obstipation	Failure to pass stool or flatus in complete obstruction
Bowel sounds	High-pitched, 'tinkling' in early obstruction; absent in late or paralytic ileus

Red flags include peritonitis, fever, tachycardia, or haemodynamic instability, which suggest ischaemia or perforation.

Pathophysiology

A bowel obstruction depends on the underlying cause, such as adhesions, hernias, volvulus, or malignancy; however, several mechanisms remain consistent across obstructive processes.

Initially, obstruction causes luminal distension. Proximal to the blockage, swallowed air, gastric secretions, and fluid produced by bacterial fermentation accumulate within the bowel. As these volumes increase, intraluminal pressure rises and stretches the bowel wall. This stimulates visceral nociceptors, resulting in the characteristic colicky abdominal pain. As pressure continues to build, venous return from the bowel wall is impaired before the arterial supply is affected. This imbalance leads to mucosal oedema and transudation of protein-rich fluid into both the bowel lumen and peritoneal cavity. The fluid sequestration that occurs contributes to hypovolaemia and electrolyte imbalance, even prior to overt vomiting.

With ongoing obstruction, peristalsis becomes impaired. The neuromuscular activity of the bowel is disrupted by progressive distension, leading to ineffective contractions and further stasis. This environment promotes bacterial overgrowth, which in turn worsens gaseous distension and fluid loss into the lumen. The cycle of stasis, overgrowth, and distension sustains the obstruction and increases the risk of bacterial translocation.

In more severe cases, particularly in closed-loop obstructions such as volvulus or a strangulated hernia, the blood supply is compromised. Venous congestion progresses to arterial insufficiency, leading to ischaemia of the bowel wall. The loss of mucosal integrity allows bacteria and endotoxins to enter the circulation, triggering systemic inflammatory responses and sepsis. If not treated promptly, the ischaemic bowel becomes necrotic, eventually perforating and causing diffuse peritonitis. Mortality rates increase significantly due to septic shock and multi-organ failure.

Vomiting and the sequestration of large volumes of fluid into the bowel and peritoneal cavity lead to severe dehydration, hypokalaemia, hyponatraemia, and often a metabolic alkalosis. As intravascular volume decreases, renal perfusion diminishes, and pre-renal acute kidney injury (AKI) may occur. In advanced cases, especially when strangulation or perforation happens, the combined effects of hypovolaemia, electrolyte imbalance, and systemic sepsis can result in circulatory collapse and shock.

Diagnosis

- History and examination: prior abdominal surgery (adhesions), hernia examination, and signs of peritonitis.
- Bloods: U&Es (dehydration), raised WCC/CRP (infection), and lactate (ischaemia).
- Imaging
  - Abdominal X-ray (AXR): dilated loops, air–fluid levels, and absence of distal gas.
  - CT abdomen/pelvis with contrast: gold standard – identifies level, cause, closed-loop, strangulation, or perforation.

Management

Initial steps

- NBM (nil by mouth).
- IV fluid resuscitation – correct hypovolaemia and electrolytes.
- Nasogastric tube (NGT) – decompress the stomach and relieve vomiting.
- Analgesia and antiemetics.
- Urinary catheterisation – monitor fluid balance.

Conservative Management

- Used for uncomplicated adhesive SBO without peritonitis.
- Serial abdominal examinations, strict input/output monitoring, and repeat imaging as needed.
- Many adhesive SBOs resolve without surgery.

Surgical Management

Indications

- Evidence of strangulation (fever, tachycardia, leucocytosis, peritonitis).
- Closed-loop obstruction.
- Perforation.
- Failure of conservative management.

Options

- Adhesiolysis.
- Bowel resection (with or without anastomosis).
- Stoma formation, depending on intraoperative findings.

Complications

- Ischaemic necrosis and perforation → peritonitis and sepsis.
- Electrolyte imbalance and AKI.
- Short bowel syndrome (after extensive resection).
- Recurrent obstruction (particularly from adhesions).

Bibliography

Catena F et al. Bowel obstruction: a review of current management strategies. World J Emerg Surg. 2019;14:20.

Fitzgibbons RJ Jr et al. Management of small bowel obstruction. N Engl J Med. 2022;386:1616–1625.

NICE. Suspected cancer: recognition and referral (NG12). 2015, updated 2023.

Royal College of Surgeons of England. Emergency General Surgery: Clinical Guidelines. 2021.

18

Bradycardias

Bradycardia is characterised by a heart rate of less than 60 beats per minute (bpm). Although this can be normal in well-conditioned individuals, such as athletes, pathological bradycardia describes an abnormally slow heart rate that causes haemodynamic instability, syncope, or end-organ hypoperfusion.

Types and Definitions

Type	Description
Sinus bradycardia	The sinus node generates impulses at <60 bpm. It may be normal (athletes) or pathological.
Sick sinus syndrome	Includes sinus pauses/arrest or brady-tachy syndrome, often due to fibrosis of the sinus node with age.
First-degree AV block	Prolonged PR interval >200 ms. Usually, benign.
Second-degree AV block	Mobitz I (Wenckebach): progressive PR prolongation, then dropped beat. Mobitz II: intermittent dropped QRS without PR change.
Third-degree AV block	Complete heart block: atria and ventricles beat independently (AV dissociation).

Causes

Intrinsic (cardiac): ischaemic heart disease, myocarditis, cardiomyopathies, Lenègre's disease (fibrosis of the conduction system), post-surgical or post-ablation damage.

Extrinsic (reversible/non-cardiac): hypothyroidism, hyperkalaemia, hypothermia, drugs (β-blockers, calcium channel blockers, digoxin, amiodarone), and increased vagal tone (Valsalva, vomiting, pain).

Pathophysiology

Bradycardias occur due to impaired impulse generation (sinus node dysfunction) or impulse conduction (AV block). Fibrosis, ischaemia, or infiltration (amyloidosis, sarcoidosis) can disrupt the conduction pathways, slowing or blocking signal transmission. In complete heart block, atrial impulses fail to reach the ventricles, which then depend on a slower, unreliable escape rhythm from junctional or ventricular foci. The resulting reduction in ventricular rate decreases cardiac output, while loss of atrial contraction further reduces ventricular filling, leading to hypotension, cerebral hypoperfusion, syncope, and heart failure symptoms.

Management

Treatment varies depending on the severity of the condition, its symptoms, and the underlying cause.

Immediate action (if haemodynamically unstable)

- Follow the ALS bradycardia algorithm (Resuscitation Council UK, 2021).
- Atropine 500 mcg IV, repeat every 3–5 min to max 3 mg.
- If ineffective
  - Transcutaneous pacing.
  - IV isoprenaline (5 mcg/min) or adrenaline (2–10 mcg/min) infusion.
  - Consider theophylline (e.g. in post-heart transplant).
  - Prepare for transvenous pacing.

Reversible Causes

- Stop rate-limiting drugs.
- Correct electrolyte imbalances (K^+, Ca^{2+}, Mg^{2+}).
- Treat hypothyroidism, hypothermia, or ischaemia/infection.

Definitive Management

A permanent pacemaker is indicated for

- Symptomatic bradycardia not correctable by reversible measures.
- Mobitz II or third-degree AV block.
- Sinus node dysfunction with significant symptoms.
- Asystolic pauses >3 seconds.

Bibliography

Kusumoto FM, Schoenfeld MH, Barrett C, et al. 2018 ACC/AHA/HRS guideline on the evaluation and management of patients with bradycardia and cardiac conduction delay. J Am Coll Cardiol. 2019;74(7):e51–e156.

National Institute for Health and Care Excellence (NICE). Cardiac arrhythmias: diagnosis and management [NG208]. 2021.

Resuscitation Council UK. Adult advanced life support guidelines. 2021.

19

Breath Sounds

Auscultation of the chest is a vital clinical skill for evaluating respiratory issues. Using the diaphragm of the stethoscope, systematically examine the chest in anterior, lateral, and posterior positions, comparing corresponding areas on each side. The patient should be asked to take slow, deep breaths through the mouth to improve sound transmission.

Normal Breath Sounds

- Vesicular: soft, low-pitched sounds heard across most of the lung fields. Inspiration lasts longer than expiration, with no pause between the two phases. These are the normal sounds of healthy lungs.
- Bronchial: harsh, loud sounds where inspiration and expiration are of similar length, separated by a pause. Typically heard over the trachea; if heard peripherally, it indicates lung consolidation (e.g. pneumonia).

Abnormal Breath Sounds

- Diminished or absent.
- Quiet breath sounds: reduced air entry may indicate pneumothorax or pleural effusion.
- Reduced/muffled sounds: often due to consolidation, collapse, or pleural effusion.

Added Sounds

- Wheeze: high-pitched, musical sounds, usually expiratory, caused by narrowed airways. Typical of asthma and chronic obstructive pulmonary disease (COPD).
- Stridor: high-pitched inspiratory sound due to upper airway obstruction (e.g. laryngeal oedema, foreign body). This is an emergency finding.
- Coarse crackles: low-pitched, popping sounds associated with retained secretions or airway collapse/reopening. Common in COPD, pneumonia, and bronchiectasis.
- Fine crackles: high-pitched, discontinuous sounds likened to Velcro being pulled apart. Often heard in pulmonary fibrosis or left ventricular failure.

- Pleural rub: harsh, grating sound due to inflamed pleural surfaces rubbing against each other. Typical of pleuritis and sometimes pneumonia.

Clinical Application

Breath sounds should always be interpreted in the context of the patient's medical history, physical examination, and imaging results. For example

- Absent sounds + hyperresonance → pneumothorax.
- Bronchial breathing + crackles → consolidation (pneumonia).
- Wheeze + polyphonic expiratory sounds → asthma/COPD.

Bibliography

British Thoracic Society. BTS clinical examination in respiratory medicine. 2020.
Epstein SK et al. Auscultation of the respiratory system. N Engl J Med. 2018;379:478–487.
NICE. Asthma: diagnosis, monitoring and chronic asthma management [NG80]. 2022.

20

Bronchoscopy

Bronchoscopy is a diagnostic and therapeutic procedure that uses a flexible fibre-optic scope passed through the mouth, nose, or endotracheal tube to visualise the trachea, bronchi, and segmental airways directly in ventilated patients. It can be performed via the endotracheal tube or tracheostomy, with appropriate monitoring and sedation according to local policy.

Indications

- Diagnostic: sampling secretions or bronchoalveolar lavage (BAL) to identify infection; assessment of airway anatomy; and biopsy of endobronchial lesions.
- Therapeutic: clearance of mucus plugs or secretions to re-expand collapsed lung regions; removal of inhaled foreign bodies; and evaluation and management of airway bleeding.
- Airway management: used as an adjunct under challenging intubations for direct visualisation.

Complications

- Bleeding: minor trauma to the mucosa is common; usually self-limiting.
- Hypoxia: transient desaturation may occur due to partial obstruction; supplemental oxygen should always be given.
- Bronchospasm: airway narrowing during the procedure, treatable with inhaled β2-agonists.
- Infection or fever: occasionally occurs after BAL or biopsy.

Airway Anatomy (Key Landmarks)

A simplified outline of the tracheobronchial tree

- Trachea → bifurcates at the carina into right and left main bronchi.
- Right main bronchus: shorter, wider, and more vertical, making it more prone to aspiration.
  - Right upper lobe bronchus
  - Right middle lobe bronchus
  - Right lower lobe bronchus
- Left main bronchus: longer and more horizontal.
  - Left upper lobe bronchus
  - Left lower lobe bronchus

Bibliography

British Thoracic Society. Guidelines for diagnostic flexible bronchoscopy in adults. Thorax. 2013;68(Suppl 1):i1–i44.

NICE. Lung Cancer: Diagnosis and Management [NG122]. 2021.

Wahidi MM et al. Technical aspects of flexible bronchoscopy. Clin Chest Med. 2018;39(1):1–16.

21

Burns Management

Burn injuries can lead to considerable morbidity and mortality because of loss of skin integrity, fluid shifts, infection risk, and systemic inflammatory responses. Prompt assessment and proper management are crucial to optimise outcomes.

Assessment of Burns

The extent and severity of burns are evaluated based on the total body surface area (TBSA) involved, the depth of the burn, the presence of inhalational injury, and any associated comorbidities.

Estimating Burn Size

- Rule of nines: the body surface is divided into areas approximately representing 9% each (e.g. each arm 9%, each leg 18%, anterior trunk 18%, posterior trunk 18%, head 9%, perineum 1%).
- Lund and Browder chart: more accurate, especially in children, as it adjusts for body proportion.

Burn Severity Classification

Minor Burns

- Adults <15% TBSA, no significant comorbidities.
- Children or elderly <10% TBSA.

Moderate Burns

- 15–30% TBSA in adults, 10–20% in the elderly.
- Any burn requiring surgical or complex wound management.
- Minor burns with significant comorbidities.

Severe Burns

- 30% TBSA in adults, >20% in the elderly.
- Inhalational injury.
- Burns associated with multiple comorbidities.
- Circumferential limb burns (risk of compartment syndrome).
- Electrical or chemical burns.
- Burns with associated trauma.

Primary Survey (A–E Approach)

Airway

- Assess for airway compromise (facial burns, soot in mouth/nose, stridor, hoarseness, singed nasal hairs).
- Early intubation is recommended if airway injury is suspected, as swelling can rapidly make intubation impossible.
- 100% oxygen should be given immediately.

Breathing

- Assess for chest wall burns that may restrict ventilation.
- Monitor oxygen saturations and consider carboxyhaemoglobin levels in suspected smoke inhalation (standard SpO_2 may be misleading).
- Treat carbon monoxide poisoning with high-flow oxygen; hyperbaric oxygen may be considered in severe cases.

Circulation

- Establish IV access (large-bore cannulae in non-burnt skin where possible).
- Burns can cause major fluid shifts due to capillary leak. Hypovolaemic shock may develop rapidly.
- Use the Parkland formula to guide fluid resuscitation.
  - 4 mL × body weight (kg) × %TBSA burn.
  - Half given in the first 8 hours from the time of burn, remainder over the next 16 hours.
- Ringer's lactate is preferred for resuscitation.
- Urinary catheterisation should be performed to monitor urine output (target 0.5–1 mL/kg/hr in adults).

Fluid Resuscitation Example

Parkland formula:

$$4\,\text{mL} \times \text{body weight}\left(\text{kg}\right) \times \%\,\text{TBSA burn}$$

Example

- 70 kg adult.
- 20% TBSA partial-thickness burn.

Calculation

$$4 \times 70 \times 20 = 5{,}600\,\text{mL over the first 24 hours}$$

- 2,800 mL in the first 8 hours (from the time of injury, not hospital admission).
- 2,800 mL in the following 16 hours.

Key Point

Fluids are only a guideline – resuscitation should always be adjusted based on urine output (0.5–1 mL/kg/hr in adults).

Secondary Survey

Disability

- Assess for associated trauma, head injury, or carbon monoxide-related neurological impairment.

Exposure

- Remove clothing/jewellery.
- Keep the patient warm; extensive burns increase the risk of hypothermia.
- Document burn depth (superficial, partial-thickness, full-thickness).

Ongoing Management

Analgesia

- IV opioids are often required; avoid IM due to unreliable absorption.
- Regular pain assessment is essential.

Wound Care

- Irrigate chemical burns with copious water (minimum 20–30 minutes).
- Debride loose non-viable tissue.
- Cover wounds with cling film or sterile sheets to reduce contamination and fluid loss.
- Avoid topical creams in the acute phase until specialist review.

Referral Criteria

Patients should be referred to a specialist burns unit if they have

- 10% TBSA in children, >15% in adults.
- Burns of face, hands, perineum, feet, or circumferential burns.
- Electrical or chemical burns.
- Inhalational injury.
- Associated trauma or comorbidities complicating management.

Complications

- Hypovolaemic shock: due to massive fluid loss.
- Infection and sepsis: skin barrier loss predisposes to infection.
- Contractures and scarring: long-term functional and cosmetic complications.
- Compartment syndrome: in circumferential limb burns.
- Multi-organ failure: due to systemic inflammatory response in major burns.

Bibliography

Advanced Trauma Life Support (ATLS®). Student Course Manual. 10th ed. American College of Surgeons; 2018.

British Burn Association. National burn care standards. 2018.

Hettiaratchy S, Papini R. Initial management of a major burn: II—assessment and resuscitation. BMJ. 2004;329:101–103.

National Institute for Health and Care Excellence (NICE). Burns and scalds: assessment and management. Clinical Knowledge Summaries. 2023.

22

Cardiac Biomarkers

Cardiac biomarkers are substances released into the bloodstream when the heart is injured or under stress. They are mainly used to support the diagnosis, risk assessment, and monitoring of acute coronary syndromes (ACS) and other heart-related conditions.

Key Biomarkers and Their Clinical Use

Biomarker	Source	Key Use	Time to Rise	Peak	Return to Normal
Troponin	Cardiac myocytes	Gold standard for MI	3–6 hrs	12–24 hrs	7–14 days
Creatine kinase (CK-MB)	Cardiac muscle (less specific than troponin)	Reinfarction detection (shorter half-life)	3–6 hrs	12–24 hrs	2–3 days
Myoglobin	Skeletal and cardiac muscle	Early marker, low specificity	1–2 hrs	6–9 hrs	<24 hrs
B-type natriuretic peptide (BNP)	Ventricles (response to stretch)	Diagnosis and monitoring of heart failure	1–4 hrs	12–24 hrs	1–2 days
High-sensitivity C-reactive protein (hs-CRP)	Liver (systemic inflammation)	Risk stratification in atherosclerosis	6 hrs	48 hrs	Variable

Troponin

Troponin is a protein complex essential to the contractile machinery of cardiac muscle cells, regulating calcium-mediated interactions between actin and myosin filaments during contraction. When myocardial injury occurs, such as during ischaemia or infarction, troponin is released into the bloodstream due to damage to cardiac myocyte membranes.

Troponin measurement is the gold standard for diagnosing acute myocardial infarction (AMI) due to its high sensitivity and specificity, enabling the detection of even minor cardiac injuries. Troponin levels

- Rise within 3–6 hours after injury.
- Peak at 12–24 hours.
- Remain elevated for 7–14 days.

This makes it valuable for both early and retrospective diagnosis.

Other Clinical Contexts

Troponin can also be elevated in

- Myocarditis
- Heart failure
- Pulmonary embolism
- Renal failure

Serial troponin measurements help distinguish between acute injury (characterised by rising or falling levels) and chronic elevations (characterised by stable but consistently high levels).

Creatine Kinase (CK and CK-MB)

Creatine kinase is an intracellular enzyme present in skeletal and cardiac muscle. The CK-MB isoenzyme is more specific to the myocardium and was traditionally utilised to diagnose myocardial infarction. However, its application has largely been replaced by troponin due to its lower sensitivity and specificity. Nonetheless, CK-MB may still be valuable in identifying reinfarction because of its shorter half-life.

Myoglobin

Myoglobin is a small, oxygen-binding protein that is released quickly from damaged muscle tissue. It increases within 1–3 hours after myocardial injury, serving as an early but non-specific marker of infarction. Elevated levels are also seen in skeletal muscle trauma, which limits its diagnostic usefulness. Its primary role is in early rule-out strategies when used in conjunction with other biomarkers.

B-Type Natriuretic Peptide (BNP) and NT-proBNP

Ventricular myocytes secrete B-type natriuretic peptide (BNP) and its inactive fragment NT-proBNP in response to increased wall stretch and volume overload. They are useful biomarkers in the diagnosis and prognosis of heart failure, correlating with disease severity and outcomes. Elevated levels may also be observed in ACSs and other conditions causing cardiac strain.

High-Sensitivity C-Reactive Protein (hs-CRP)

High-sensitivity C-reactive protein (hs-CRP) is an acute-phase reactant produced by the liver in response to systemic inflammation. Although not specific to cardiac injury, elevated hs-CRP has prognostic value in cardiovascular disease. It indicates vascular inflammation and is linked to a higher risk of atherosclerosis, acute coronary events, and worse outcomes after myocardial infarction.

Bibliography

Collet J-P et al. 2020 ESC Guidelines for the management of acute coronary syndromes in patients presenting without persistent ST-segment elevation. Eur Heart J. 2021;42:1289–1367.

Maisel A et al. Biomarkers in heart failure. N Engl J Med. 2011;365:2557–2566.

NICE. Chest pain of recent onset: assessment and diagnosis [CG95]. 2023 update.

Thygesen K et al. Fourth universal definition of myocardial infarction (2018). Eur Heart J. 2019;40(3):237–269.

23

Cardiac Output Studies

Cardiac output (CO) refers to the volume of blood the heart pumps per minute and is a vital measure of cardiac function and overall blood flow. Sufficient CO is necessary for supplying oxygen and nutrients to tissues, and monitoring CO offers essential insights into critically ill patients.

Formula:

$$CO = SV \times HR$$

- Stroke volume (SV): the amount of blood ejected by the left ventricle with each contraction.
- Heart rate (HR): the number of beats per minute.

Measurement Techniques

1) Invasive methods
   - Thermodilution via pulmonary artery catheter (Swan–Ganz catheter): the most commonly used invasive method. A known volume of cold saline is injected into the right atrium, and a thermistor in the pulmonary artery detects temperature fluctuations. The change in temperature over time is used to determine CO. This technique allows for continuous monitoring but involves risks such as arrhythmia, thrombosis, and infection.
   - Dye and indicator dilution methods: involve injecting a dye (e.g. indocyanine green) or an inert indicator into the bloodstream and analysing its downstream concentration curve. Less frequently employed due to complexity and the availability of alternative techniques.
2) Non-invasive methods
   - Doppler ultrasound: uses ultrasound waves to measure blood flow velocity in the aorta or pulmonary artery. Combined with vessel diameter, it estimates SV and CO. Useful in perioperative and critical care settings.
   - Bioimpedance and bioreactance: these methods measure thoracic electrical impedance or phase shifts caused by cardiac cycles, offering a continuous estimate of CO.

They are non-invasive and portable but may be less accurate in patients with fluid shifts, arrhythmias, or pulmonary oedema.
- Echocardiography: a widely accessible and non-invasive tool. SV is determined using the left ventricular outflow tract (LVOT) area and the velocity time integral (VTI) of blood flow. It offers additional information on cardiac structure, contractility, and filling pressures.

Determinants of CO

1) Preload
   - End-diastolic volume in the ventricles.
   - Governed by venous return.
   - Increased preload usually increases CO (Frank–Starling mechanism) until a plateau is reached.
2) Afterload
   - The resistance the ventricle must overcome to eject blood.
   - Increased afterload (e.g. systemic hypertension, aortic stenosis) reduces CO.
3) Contractility
   - The intrinsic ability of the myocardium to contract independently of preload and afterload.
   - Influenced by sympathetic activity, myocardial health, and inotropic drugs.
4) Heart rate
   - Moderate increases raise CO, but excessive tachycardia reduces diastolic filling time and SV, impairing output.

Clinical Relevance

- In heart failure, CO is decreased due to impaired contractility or abnormal preload and afterload relationships.
- In shock states (e.g. hypovolaemic, cardiogenic, distributive), CO monitoring assists in guiding fluid therapy, vasopressor administration, and inotropic support.
- In sepsis, CO may initially rise (hyperdynamic state) but later decrease due to myocardial depression and poor perfusion.

Monitoring CO enables clinicians to adjust interventions and optimise oxygen delivery (DO_2), particularly in critical care and perioperative medicine.

Limitations and Considerations

- Invasive methods offer accuracy but pose risks such as infection, vascular injury, arrhythmias, and pulmonary artery rupture (rare but catastrophic).
- Non-invasive methods are safer and easier to use but may be less reliable in unstable patients with arrhythmias, obesity, or fluid shifts.

- Measurements should always be interpreted within the context of the patient's overall haemodynamic condition, rather than in isolation.
- Dynamic assessment (e.g. response to fluids, passive leg raise test) often yields more helpful information than a static CO value.

Bibliography

Guyton AC, Hall JE. Textbook of Medical Physiology. 14th ed. Elsevier; 2021.

Monnet X, Teboul J-L. Assessment of cardiac output in critically ill patients. Eur Heart J. 2017;38(47):3706–3717.

National Institute for Health and Care Excellence (NICE). Haemodynamic monitoring in critical care. 2022.

Vincent JL, De Backer D. Circulatory shock. N Engl J Med. 2013;369:1726–1734.

24

Cardiac Surgeries Overview

This chapter offers a brief overview of common cardiac surgeries. It aims to highlight key procedures and general principles but does not cover the full range of surgical techniques, detailed indications, or post-operative management.

Coronary Artery Bypass Grafting (CABG)

Coronary artery bypass grafting (CABG) is performed in patients with significant coronary artery disease that causes myocardial ischaemia or infarction. Conduits, such as the saphenous vein or internal mammary artery, are harvested and grafted to bypass blocked coronary arteries, thereby restoring blood flow to the myocardium.

Goals

- Relieve angina.
- Improve myocardial oxygenation.
- Reduce risk of further cardiac damage.
- Improve survival in selected patients (e.g. left main disease, triple-vessel disease).

CABG remains a key treatment for patients unsuitable for percutaneous coronary intervention (PCI) or with complex coronary anatomy.

Valve Repair or Replacement

Heart valve surgery is undertaken when severe valvular disease causes symptoms, left ventricular dysfunction, or risk of sudden deterioration. The two main surgical strategies are valve repair and valve replacement.

Valve Repair

Where feasible, repair is preferred because it preserves the native valve and maintains more physiological function. Mitral valve repair is commonly used in the treatment of degenerative mitral regurgitation, employing techniques such as annuloplasty rings or leaflet reconstruction. Repair reduces the risk of prosthesis-related complications and often avoids the need for long-term anticoagulation.

Valve Replacement

When repair is not feasible, the diseased valve is replaced with either a mechanical or a biological (tissue) prosthesis.

- Mechanical valves are constructed from durable materials such as carbon and titanium. They have excellent longevity, often lasting for decades, making them suitable for younger patients. However, they are thrombogenic and require lifelong anticoagulation with warfarin to prevent valve thrombosis and systemic embolism. This necessitates regular International Normalised Ratio monitoring and carries a risk of bleeding complications.
- Tissue valves are made from porcine, bovine, or human donor tissue. Their main benefit is that they usually do not require long-term anticoagulation, except for a short course after surgery, unless other factors suggest otherwise. They are often chosen for older patients or those who cannot take anticoagulation. The primary disadvantage is limited durability, with structural valve degeneration typically occurring after 10–20 years, and sometimes sooner in younger patients.

Anticoagulation Considerations

The choice between mechanical and tissue valves involves weighing the risks of anticoagulation against the durability of the valve. Shared decision-making with patients is essential, considering age, comorbidities, lifestyle, and preferences. Novel oral anticoagulants (NOACs/DOACs) are not recommended for patients with mechanical valves, making warfarin the standard treatment.

Congenital Heart Defect Repair

Congenital heart disease covers a broad spectrum of structural abnormalities present from birth. Surgical intervention is often necessary to restore standard cardiac structure, improve haemodynamics, and boost long-term survival and quality of life. Progress in paediatric cardiac surgery and perioperative care has significantly improved outcomes, with many patients now living well into adulthood.

Commonly treated defects

- Atrial septal defects (ASDs) and ventricular septal defects (VSDs): surgical or catheter-based closure prevents left-to-right shunting, which otherwise causes right heart dilatation, arrhythmias, and pulmonary hypertension. Early correction reduces long-term complications such as atrial fibrillation and right-sided heart failure.
- Tetralogy of Fallot: repair generally involves closing the VSD and relieving right ventricular outflow tract obstruction. Surgery restores near-normal oxygen levels and reduces cyanotic spells, significantly improving survival.

- Transposition of the great arteries (TGAs): this condition, in which the aorta and pulmonary artery are transposed, is incompatible with life without treatment. The arterial switch operation is now the standard repair, restoring regular ventriculo-arterial connections and supporting long-term outcomes.
- Complex malformations: conditions such as hypoplastic left heart syndrome often require staged surgical palliation (e.g. Norwood, Glenn, and Fontan procedures), rather than definitive repair. These operations aim to optimise circulation and improve functional capacity, although long-term complications remain common.

Benefits of Early Intervention

Timely surgery enhances systemic oxygen delivery, decreases cyanosis, and prevents the progression of irreversible pulmonary vascular disease. It also lowers the risk of arrhythmias, ventricular dysfunction, and heart failure later in life. Psychosocial outcomes, including growth and development in children, are also improved by early correction.

Lifelong Considerations

Even after successful repair, patients often need long-term follow-up. Residual shunts, valve issues, arrhythmias, and heart failure may develop years after surgery. Many adults with repaired congenital defects are now cared for in specialist adult congenital heart disease (ACHD) clinics, highlighting the need for ongoing monitoring and multidisciplinary management.

Heart Transplantation

Heart transplantation is the definitive treatment for patients with end-stage heart failure who remain symptomatic despite maximum medical therapy, device implantation, or surgical revascularisation. Advances in surgical techniques, immunosuppression, and perioperative care have established transplantation as a reliable treatment, providing both extended survival and significant improvements in quality of life.

Indications

The most common indications include advanced heart failure caused by ischaemic cardiomyopathy, dilated cardiomyopathy, or congenital heart disease. Patients may be considered for treatment when optimal pharmacological therapy (including angiotensin-converting enzyme [ACE] inhibitors, beta-blockers, mineralocorticoid receptor antagonists, and sodium-glucose co-transporter 2 [SGLT2] inhibitors) fails to manage symptoms, and when alternative interventions such as ventricular assist devices (VADs), implantable cardioverter-defibrillators (ICDs), or revascularisation are no longer effective. Careful patient selection is crucial, as transplantation necessitates lifelong adherence to immunosuppressive regimens and ongoing long-term follow-up.

The Procedure

The operation involves removing the diseased native heart and implanting a donor heart. Donor organs are generally retrieved from brainstem-dead individuals with no significant cardiac disease. Time is critical, as cold ischaemic time (the period between organ retrieval and implantation) directly affects graft survival. In the operating theatre, the patient is placed on cardiopulmonary bypass while the diseased heart is excised, leaving a cuff of the atria and great vessels. The donor heart is then connected to these structures, restoring circulation once the graft is re-perfused.

Immunosuppression and Rejection

Lifelong immunosuppressive therapy is crucial to prevent graft rejection. Typical regimens involve a combination of calcineurin inhibitors (e.g. tacrolimus or cyclosporine), antiproliferative agents (such as mycophenolate mofetil or azathioprine), and corticosteroids. Rejection can be hyperacute, acute, or chronic.

- Acute rejection is most common in the first year and is monitored by endomyocardial biopsy and echocardiography.
- Chronic rejection, also termed cardiac allograft vasculopathy, manifests as diffuse coronary artery disease and remains a major cause of late graft loss.

Outcomes and Prognosis

Despite the challenges of donor availability and complications from long-term immunosuppression, transplantation provides significant benefits. The median survival after heart transplantation now exceeds 12 years, with many patients living considerably longer. Most recipients see a dramatic improvement in exercise tolerance, functional capacity, and quality of life compared to their pre-transplant condition.

Complications

Long-term management is primarily influenced by the risks associated with immunosuppression. These include heightened vulnerability to infection, renal impairment (especially from calcineurin inhibitors), metabolic issues such as diabetes and hypertension, and malignancies like skin cancers and post-transplant lymphoproliferative disease. Graft vasculopathy remains a unique and significant late complication, requiring monitoring with angiography or intravascular imaging.

Donor Availability and Ethical Considerations

The donor shortage remains the biggest challenge, with demand significantly exceeding supply. This has resulted in an increased use of mechanical circulatory support, especially left ventricular assist devices (LVADs), as either a bridge to transplantation or as long-term treatment for patients who are unsuitable for transplantation. Ethical issues related to donor consent, allocation of limited organs, and fair access continue to be key concerns in transplantation programmes worldwide.

Bibliography

Erbel R et al. 2014 ESC Guidelines on the diagnosis and treatment of aortic diseases. Eur Heart J. 2014;35:2873–2926.

Neumann FJ et al. 2018 ESC/EACTS Guidelines on myocardial revascularization. Eur Heart J. 2019;40(2):87–165.

Otto CM, Nishimura RA, Bonow RO, et al. 2020 ACC/AHA guideline for the management of patients with valvular heart disease. J Am Coll Cardiol. 2021;77(4):e25–e197.

Ross HJ et al. The International Society for Heart and Lung Transplantation Guidelines for the care of heart transplant recipients. J Heart Lung Transplant. 2010;29(8):914–956.

25

Cardiac Tamponade

Cardiac tamponade is a life-threatening condition caused by the build-up of fluid (blood, pus, serous fluid, or gas) in the pericardial sac, which increases intrapericardial pressure. This hampers ventricular filling and decreases cardiac output. The condition may develop suddenly (e.g. trauma) or gradually (e.g. malignancy, infection).

Causes

Category	Examples
Trauma	Penetrating wounds (stab, gunshot), blunt trauma, and cardiac surgery
Malignancy	Lung, breast, lymphoma, and metastatic disease
Infection	Viral pericarditis (e.g. coxsackievirus), TB, and bacterial pericarditis
Iatrogenic	Cardiac catheterisation, pacemaker insertion, and central line placement
Autoimmune/ inflammatory	SLE, rheumatoid arthritis, and Dressler's syndrome
Uraemia	End-stage renal disease
Aortic dissection	Rupture into the pericardial sac
Hypothyroidism	Can cause pericardial effusion
Radiation	Radiation-induced pericarditis

Pathophysiology

The pericardium typically handles the gradual accumulation of fluid of up to 1–2 L, but a sudden accumulation of just 100–200 mL can be fatal.

1) Increased intrapericardial pressure: as fluid accumulates, pericardial pressure rises. Once this exceeds right atrial and ventricular diastolic pressures, ventricular filling becomes restricted.
2) Impaired ventricular filling: reduced preload results in decreased stroke volume and cardiac output, initially compensated by tachycardia.

3) Ventricular interdependence: right-sided compression shifts the septum leftward, decreasing LV filling during inspiration. This explains pulsus paradoxus (a fall in SBP > 10 mmHg on inspiration).
4) Failure of compensation: sympathetic stimulation initially maintains perfusion, but progressive tamponade results in hypotension, shock, and cardiac arrest.

Clinical Features

Classic (Beck's triad)

- Hypotension (low stroke volume)
- Elevated jugular venous pressure (JVP) (impaired venous return)
- Muffled heart sounds (fluid insulation)

Other findings

- Pulsus paradoxus
- Tachycardia and dyspnoea
- Narrow pulse pressure
- ECG: electrical alternans and low QRS voltage
- CXR: 'Water bottle' heart (subacute cases)
- Echocardiography: diastolic collapse of right atrium/ventricle (gold standard)

Management

- Emergency pericardiocentesis: definitive, ultrasound-guided drainage relieves intrapericardial pressure and restores cardiac filling.
- Trauma-induced tamponade: an urgent thoracotomy might be necessary.
- Recurrent or permanent management: pericardial window or treatment of the underlying cause (malignancy, infection, autoimmune disease).

Bibliography

Adler Y, Charron P, Imazio M, et al. 2015 ESC Guidelines for the diagnosis and management of pericardial diseases. Eur Heart J. 2015;36(42):2921–2964.

Ristić AD, Imazio M, Adler Y, et al. Triage strategy for urgent management of cardiac tamponade: a position statement of the European Society of Cardiology. Eur Heart J. 2014;35(34):2279–2284.

Spodick DH. Acute cardiac tamponade. N Engl J Med. 2003;349(7):684–690.

26

Cerebrospinal Fluid Analysis

Cerebrospinal fluid (CSF) analysis is a crucial diagnostic tool in evaluating central nervous system (CNS) disorders. By examining the physical, chemical, and cellular components of CSF, clinicians can identify infections, inflammatory conditions, malignancies, and other neurological pathologies.

Typical CSF Findings

Parameter	Normal CSF	Bacterial Meningitis	Viral Meningitis	TB Meningitis	Subarachnoid Haemorrhage (SAH)
Appearance	Clear	Turbid/ cloudy	Clear or slightly cloudy	Faintly cloudy/ yellow	Bloody or xanthochromia
Opening pressure	10–20 cm H_2O	↑ (>30 cm H_2O)	Normal or ↑	↑	↑
WCC (/x 10^9/L)	<5 (mostly lymphocytes)	↑↑ (10–50, neutrophils)	↑ (1–10, lymphocytes)	↑ (5–50, lymphocytes)	Normal or mildly ↑
Differential cells	Lymphocytes	Neutrophils	Lymphocytes	Lymphocytes	RBCs predominate
Protein (g/L)	0.15–0.45	↑↑ (1–5)	Mild ↑ (0.5–1)	↑↑ (very high)	Mild ↑
Glucose (mmol/L)	2.5–4.4	↓ (<2.2 or < 50% serum)	Normal or mildly ↓	↓	Normal
CSF: serum glucose ratio	>0.6	<0.4	>0.5	<0.4	Normal
Gram stain	Negative	Often positive	Negative	Negative	Negative
Culture	Negative	Usually positive	Usually negative	May grow *Mycobacterium tuberculosis*	Negative
Special tests	—	—	—	Acid fast Bacilli (AFB) stain, PCR, culture	Xanthochromia, RBCs not clearing

Diagnostic Patterns

- Bacterial meningitis → high neutrophils + ↓ glucose + very high protein.
- Viral meningitis → high lymphocytes + normal glucose.
- Tuberculous meningitis → high lymphocytes + ↓ glucose + very high protein.
- Subarachnoid haemorrhage (SAH) → xanthochromia + persistent RBCs.

Bibliography

Hasbun, R. (2025) Clinical features and diagnosis of acute bacterial meningitis in adults. In: Tunkel, A.R. and White, N. (eds.) UpToDate. Available at: https://www.uptodate.com/contents/clinical-features-and-diagnosis-of-acutebacterial-meningitis-in-adults

National Institute for Health and Care Excellence (NICE). Bacterial meningitis and meningococcal septicaemia in children and young people (NG143). 2021.

Solomon T, Michael BD, Smith PE, et al. Management of suspected viral encephalitis in adults – Association of British Neurologists and British Infection Association national guideline. J Infect. 2012;64(4):347–373.

Tunkel AR, van de Beek D, Scheld WM. Acute meningitis. N Engl J Med. 2021;384:54–63.

27

Chest X-Ray Interpretation

A chest X-ray (CXR) is a fundamental diagnostic tool in critical care and general clinical practice, providing information on the lungs, heart, mediastinum, pleura, and chest wall. A systematic approach avoids missed findings. The most widely used method in UK practice is RIPE–ABCDE.

Step 1: Confirm Details – RIPE

Component	Description
R – rotation	Clavicles equidistant from spinous processes
I – inspiration	5–6 anterior ribs visible above the diaphragm
P – penetration	Vertebrae are just visible behind the heart
E – exposure/ identification	Correct patient, date, and view. PA = standard; AP = ITU/immobile patients (magnifies heart)

Step 2: Systematic Review – ABCDE

Step	What to Check	Key Points and Common Pathologies
A – airway/ mediastinum	Trachea central? Mediastinal contours	Deviation = collapse, mass, and tension pneumothorax
B – breathing	Compare lung fields	Consolidation, effusion, collapse, and pneumothorax
C – circulation	Heart size, aortic contour, and hila	Cardiothoracic ratio < 50% on PA
D – diaphragm	Hemidiaphragms and costophrenic angles	Blunting = effusion; free air = perforation
E – everything else	Bones, soft tissues, and devices	Fractures, lines/tubes, and foreign bodies

Normal Landmarks

Structure	Normal Appearance
Trachea	Central or slightly right
Lungs	Radiolucent and symmetrical
Heart size	<50% thoracic width (PA)
Diaphragm	Right higher than left and smooth
Costophrenic angles	Sharp and clear
Hila	Left is higher than right

Common Findings

Finding	Interpretation
Consolidation	Lobar opacity and air bronchograms → pneumonia
Collapse (atelectasis)	Loss of volume and tracheal deviation towards the side
Pleural effusion	Blunted angle, meniscus sign, and mediastinal shift
Pneumothorax	No lung markings, pleural edge, and trachea away if tension
Cardiomegaly	Heart >50% thoracic width (PA)
Pulmonary oedema	Bat-wing pattern, Kerley B lines, and cardiomegaly
Interstitial lung disease	Reticular/nodular and basal predominance
Free air	Under diaphragm → perforation

Lines and Tubes: Position Check

Device	Normal Position
ET tube	5 cm above carina (T4/5)
NG tube	Below the diaphragm, in the stomach (check locally)
Central line	Superior vena cava (SVC) near the cavo-atrial junction
Chest drain	In the pleural space, fenestrations are not outside the chest wall

Bibliography

Fraser RS, Colman N, Müller NL, Paré PD. Diagnosis of Diseases of the Chest. 4th ed. Saunders; 1999.

Talley NJ, O'Connor S. Clinical Examination: A Systematic Guide to Physical Diagnosis. 9th ed. Elsevier; 2022.

The Royal College of Radiologists. Standards for Interpretation and Reporting of Imaging Investigations. RCR; 2018.

28

Chronic Liver Disease

Chronic liver disease (CLD) refers to progressive deterioration of liver structure and function lasting longer than 6 months. It encompasses a spectrum of disorders that result in fibrosis, cirrhosis, and potentially liver failure.

Definition and Core Features

CLD is characterised by

- Persistent elevation of liver enzymes (Alanine Aminotransferase (ALT), Aspartate Aminotransferase (AST), Alkalne Phosphatase (ALP), Gamma-Glutamyl Transferase (GGT)).
- Evidence of fibrosis or cirrhosis on imaging, elastography, or biopsy.
- Clinical features such as jaundice, portal hypertension, and hepatic encephalopathy.

Causes of Chronic Liver Disease

Type	Examples
Viral hepatitis	Hepatitis B, Hepatitis C
Alcohol-related liver disease	Chronic alcohol misuse
Non-alcoholic fatty liver disease (NAFLD)	Metabolic syndrome, obesity, type 2 diabetes
Autoimmune liver diseases	Autoimmune hepatitis, primary biliary cholangitis (PBC), and primary sclerosing cholangitis (PSC)
Genetic/metabolic disorders	Hemochromatosis, Wilson's disease, and alpha-1 antitrypsin deficiency
Drug-induced liver injury	Methotrexate, amiodarone, antibiotics, and chemotherapy agents

Pathophysiology

CLD develops because of repeated or sustained injury to hepatocytes. This ongoing damage triggers an inflammatory response, which, over time, disrupts the liver's typical architecture and function.

A key step in this process is the activation of hepatic stellate cells. Under normal conditions, these cells store vitamin A and remain quiescent. Persistent hepatocellular injury, however, causes them to transform into myofibroblasts, which begin producing collagen and other extracellular matrix proteins. This excessive deposition of fibrotic tissue gradually distorts the liver parenchyma.

As fibrosis advances, the buildup of scar tissue disrupts the standard lobular architecture. The development of regenerative nodules and bridging fibrosis ultimately leads to cirrhosis, characterised by a nodular, scarred appearance of the liver and a significant loss of its functional capacity.

The architectural distortion also has significant haemodynamic effects. Increased resistance to blood flow through the diseased liver causes portal hypertension, which is key to many complications of CLD. Elevated portal pressure results in the formation of oesophageal and gastric varices, ascites due to fluid transudation, splenomegaly, and hypersplenism, leading to secondary cytopenias.

Finally, the loss of viable hepatocytes impairs the liver's synthetic and detoxifying functions. Reduced albumin production contributes to oedema and ascites, while decreased synthesis of clotting factors increases the risk of bleeding and coagulopathy. Impaired detoxification of nitrogenous waste products, particularly ammonia, leads to their accumulation in the bloodstream, resulting in hepatic encephalopathy. Together, these pathophysiological processes form the basis of the clinical signs and complications seen in advanced liver disease.

Clinical Features

- Early disease: often silent or non-specific (fatigue, malaise, anorexia).
- Progressive/decompensated disease:
  - Jaundice
  - Ascites and peripheral oedema
  - Hepatic encephalopathy (confusion, asterixis, drowsiness)
  - Variceal bleeding (from oesophageal/gastric varices due to portal hypertension)
  - Coagulopathy (easy bruising, bleeding)
  - Cutaneous signs: spider naevi, palmar erythema, caput medusae, and gynecomastia

Management

1) Address underlying cause
   - Antivirals for hepatitis B/C.
   - Abstinence, support, and pharmacotherapy for alcohol-related disease.
   - Weight loss, diabetes, and lipid control for non-alcoholic fatty liver disease (NAFLD).
   - Immunosuppressants for autoimmune hepatitis.

2) Manage complications
   - Ascites → spironolactone ± furosemide and paracentesis if refractory.
   - Varices → non-selective beta-blockers (propranolol) and endoscopic band ligation.
   - Encephalopathy → lactulose and rifaximin.
   - Coagulopathy → vitamin K and fresh frozen plasma (FFP) if bleeding.
3) Surveillance
   - Hepatocellular carcinoma screening with ultrasound ± alpha-fetoprotein (AFP) every 6 months.
   - Endoscopy for variceal screening in cirrhosis.
4) Definitive treatment
   - Liver transplantation for decompensated cirrhosis, model for end stage liver disease (MELD) > 15, or acute-on-chronic liver failure.

Prognosis

- Depends on cause, stage of fibrosis, and comorbidities.
- Tools such as the Child–Pugh score and MELD score help predict prognosis and guide transplant referral.

Bibliography

Arroyo V, Moreau R, Kamath PS, Jalan R, Ginès P. Acute-on-chronic liver failure in cirrhosis. Nat Rev Dis Primers. 2016;2:16041.

European Association for the Study of the Liver (EASL). EASL Clinical Practice Guidelines: management of chronic liver diseases. J Hepatol. 2021.

NICE NG50. Cirrhosis in Over 16s: Assessment and Management. 2016.

Tapper EB, Lok AS. Management of cirrhosis and its complications. N Engl J Med. 2017;377:817–827.

29

Chronic Obstructive Pulmonary Disease

Chronic obstructive pulmonary disease (COPD) is a common, preventable, and treatable progressive lung disease characterised by persistent airflow limitation and chronic respiratory symptoms, primarily caused by exposure to noxious particles or gases.

Diagnosis

The diagnosis of COPD relies on a combination of clinical features and objective tests. Patients often present with a chronic cough, sputum production, and increasing exertional breathlessness, which may initially be mistaken for ageing or lowered fitness. Careful history-taking is essential to identify risk factors such as smoking, occupational exposures, or a family history of respiratory disease. The key diagnostic tool, however, is spirometry, providing a quantitative measure of airflow limitation. A post-bronchodilator ratio of forced expiratory volume in one second (FEV_1) to forced vital capacity (FVC) of less than 0.7 confirms persistent airflow obstruction. Importantly, this obstruction is not fully reversible, distinguishing COPD from asthma and making spirometry crucial for diagnosis and staging.

Causes

Cause	Description
Smoking	Leading cause: damages small airways and alveoli
Environmental exposures	Biomass smoke, occupational dusts, and chemical fumes
Genetic factors	Alpha-1 antitrypsin deficiency (rare but essential in younger patients)
Other	Recurrent childhood respiratory infections

Pathophysiology

Chronic exposure to inhaled irritants (especially tobacco smoke) triggers a persistent inflammatory response involving neutrophils, macrophages, and CD8 + T lymphocytes. These cells release proteases and reactive oxygen species, leading to

- Emphysema: protease–antiprotease imbalance leads to alveolar wall destruction, reducing gas exchange surface area and elastic recoil.
- Airway remodelling: goblet cell hyperplasia, mucus hypersecretion, and fibrosis leading to chronic bronchitis and airway narrowing.
- Air trapping and hyperinflation: reduced expiratory flow caused by loss of recoil.
- Pulmonary vascular disease: endothelial dysfunction and remodelling lead to pulmonary hypertension and cor pulmonale.

Clinical Features

- Chronic productive cough.
- Progressive breathlessness (initially exertional → later at rest).
- Wheeze and chest tightness.
- Frequent infective exacerbations.
- Advanced signs: cyanosis, barrel chest, accessory muscle use, cachexia, and signs of right heart failure (raised jugular venour pressure [JVP], oedema).

Investigations

Test	Purpose
Spirometry	Confirm diagnosis and grade severity (FEV_1 % predicted)
Chest X-ray	Exclude differential diagnoses and detect hyperinflation/emphysema
Arterial blood gases	Identify hypoxaemia and hypercapnia
Alpha-1 antitrypsin levels	In younger or non-smokers with COPD
CT chest	Assess emphysema, bronchiectasis, or surgical candidacy

Management

1) Lifestyle and prevention
   - Smoking cessation (most effective intervention)
   - Vaccinations: annual influenza and pneumococcal vaccines
2) Pharmacological
   - Short-acting bronchodilators (SABA/SAMA) for relief
   - Long-acting bronchodilators (LABA/LAMA) for maintenance
   - Inhaled corticosteroids (ICS) for frequent exacerbators or eosinophilic phenotype

   - Triple therapy (LABA/LAMA/ICS) in advanced disease
3) Non-pharmacological
   - Pulmonary rehabilitation (exercise, nutrition, education)
   - Oxygen therapy: long-term (>15 hours/day) if chronic hypoxaemia ($PaO_2 \leq 7.3$ kPa, or ≤ 8 kPa with complications)
   - Nutritional support and management of comorbidities
4) Exacerbations
   - Oral corticosteroids (e.g. prednisolone 30 mg for 5 days)
   - Antibiotics if purulent sputum or bacterial infection suspected
   - Escalated bronchodilator therapy
5) Surgical options
   - Lung volume reduction surgery (selected emphysema patients)
   - Lung transplantation in end-stage disease

Prognosis

COPD is a progressive disease, but key interventions can influence its course. Smoking cessation remains the most effective measure to slow decline, while vaccination and optimised pharmacological therapy reduce exacerbations and enhance quality of life. Prognosis is often evaluated using the BODE index, which considers body mass index, degree of airflow obstruction, level of dyspnoea, and exercise capacity to provide a more accurate prediction of survival than spirometry alone. The leading causes of death in COPD include respiratory failure, right-sided heart failure, lung cancer, and cardiovascular disease, highlighting the systemic effects of the condition beyond the lungs.

Bibliography

Global Initiative for Chronic Obstructive Lung Disease (GOLD). Global strategy for diagnosis, management, and prevention of COPD. 2024 Report.

NICE NG115. Chronic obstructive pulmonary disease in over 16s: diagnosis and management. 2019.

Wedzicha JA, Seemungal TA. COPD exacerbations: defining their cause and prevention. Lancet. 2007;370(9589):786–796.

30

Coagulopathy

Coagulopathy refers to impaired blood clotting, which can present as hypocoagulability (a tendency to bleed), hypercoagulability (a risk of thrombosis), or both. It may be inherited (e.g. haemophilia, von Willebrand disease) or acquired (e.g. liver disease, vitamin K deficiency, disseminated intravascular coagulation [DIC], anticoagulant therapy).

Definition and Diagnosis

Suspicion arises from a history of bleeding, bruising, or thrombosis, confirmed by laboratory abnormalities.

- Prolonged PT/INR: extrinsic pathway and warfarin effect
- Prolonged aPTT: intrinsic pathway and heparin effect
- Low platelets: thrombocytopenia
- Low fibrinogen: DIC and massive transfusion
- Raised D-dimer: fibrinolysis/consumption

Advanced tests: factor assays and thromboelastography/rotational thromboelastometry (TEG/ROTEM).

Causes

Inherited	Acquired
Haemophilia A (VIII deficiency)	Liver disease (↓ clotting factors)
Haemophilia B (IX deficiency)	Vitamin K deficiency (↓ II, VII, IX, X)
von Willebrand disease	DIC (consumption coagulopathy)
Rare factor deficiencies	Anticoagulants (warfarin, heparin, direct oral anti-coagulant [DOACs])
	Massive transfusion/dilution
	Sepsis, trauma-induced coagulopathy

Pathophysiology

Disorders of coagulation can result in either bleeding or thrombotic states, depending on the underlying imbalance. Bleeding tendencies develop from impaired platelet function, deficiencies in clotting factors, or depletion of fibrinogen, all of which hinder the formation of an effective haemostatic clot. Conversely, thrombotic states are caused by excessive thrombin generation or impaired fibrinolysis, which lead to intravascular clot formation and a higher risk of vessel occlusion. A particularly severe condition, DIC, involves both processes: widespread microvascular thrombosis consumes clotting factors and platelets, making the patient simultaneously susceptible to bleeding and thrombosis. Liver disease further hampers haemostasis by decreasing the production of both procoagulant and anticoagulant proteins. In contrast, vitamin K deficiency impairs the γ-carboxylation of key clotting factors (II, VII, IX, and X), resulting in ineffective coagulation and an increased risk of bleeding.

Management

Treatment varies depending on the underlying cause and severity of bleeding.

- Vitamin K deficiency → vitamin K (oral/IV).
- Warfarin reversal → vitamin K + prothrombin complex concentrate (PCC) ± FFP.
- Heparin reversal → protamine sulphate.
- DIC → treat cause, supportive replacement (FFP, cryoprecipitate, platelets).
- Trauma/major bleeding → massive transfusion protocol (1:1:1 PRBC:FFP:platelets).
- Hypofibrinogenemia → cryoprecipitate/fibrinogen concentrate.
- Haemophilia → recombinant factor VIII or IX.
- von Willebrand disease → desmopressin (DDAVP) or von Willebrand factor (vWF) concentrates.

Bibliography

Hunt BJ. Bleeding and coagulopathies in critical care. N Engl J Med. 2014;370:847–859.
Levi M et al. Disseminated intravascular coagulation. N Engl J Med. 2018;379:1245–1256.
NICE NG24. Blood transfusion. 2015.

31

Common Head Injuries

Head injuries vary from mild concussions to severe intracranial haemorrhages. Their impact depends on the injury mechanism, the amount of bleeding, and the increase in intracranial pressure (ICP). Early recognition and treatment are crucial in reducing morbidity and mortality.

Types of Head Injury

Concussion

- Mild traumatic brain injury caused by sudden acceleration or deceleration.
- Pathophysiology: neuronal dysfunction caused by ionic shifts, glutamate release, and altered neurotransmission.
- Clinical: transient confusion, amnesia, headache, and dizziness, with no structural damage evident on imaging.

Contusion

- Localised brain bruise with capillary bleeding and oedema.
- May be coup (at impact site) or contrecoup (opposite site).
- Can cause focal neurological deficits depending on location.

Epidural Haematoma

- Commonly from a temporal bone fracture, tearing the middle meningeal artery.
- Arterial bleed between skull and dura → rapid ICP rise.
- Classic 'lucid interval' before rapid deterioration.
- Urgent neurosurgical evacuation is often required.

Subdural Haematoma

- Tearing of bridging veins between the dura mater and the brain surface.
- Slower venous bleed → gradual ICP rise.
- Acute form after trauma; chronic form develops over weeks in elderly/anticoagulated patients.

Subarachnoid Haemorrhage

- Bleeding into the subarachnoid space from ruptured vessels.
- Causes meningeal irritation, raised ICP, and risk of vasospasm.
- May coexist with other traumatic intracranial injuries.

Management Principles

- Initial assessment: airway, breathing, circulation (ABCs) and cervical spine protection.
- Neurological assessment: Glasgow Coma Scale (GCS), pupil size and reactivity, and limb responses.
- Imaging: non-contrast CT head to evaluate suspected intracranial injury.
- ICP control: elevate head 30°, sedation, and osmotic therapy (mannitol or hypertonic saline).
- Surgical intervention: evacuation of epidural or subdural haematoma; decompressive craniectomy if ICP is raised.
- Supportive care: analgesia, seizure prophylaxis, maintenance of normotension, and avoiding hypoxia and hypotension.
- Observation: mild injuries might only necessitate monitoring and relief of symptoms.

Bibliography

Bullock MR et al. Guidelines for the management of severe traumatic brain injury. J Neurotrauma. 2007;24(Suppl 1):S1–S106.

Carney N et al. Traumatic brain injury management update. Lancet Neurol. 2017;16(4):311–322.

NICE CG176. Head injury: assessment and early management. 2017.

32

Delirium

Delirium is an acute, fluctuating disturbance in attention, awareness, and cognition that develops over hours to days. It is a clinical syndrome characterised by sudden brain dysfunction, especially affecting the reticular activating system and the prefrontal cortex.

Causes

Delirium is typically multifactorial, resulting from a combination of underlying vulnerability (such as age, dementia, sensory impairment) and acute precipitating factors.

- Drugs: anticholinergics, opioids, benzodiazepines, and polypharmacy.
- Infections: pneumonia, urinary tract infection, and sepsis.
- Metabolic: hyponatraemia, hypoglycaemia, and renal or hepatic failure.
- Withdrawal: alcohol or sedatives.
- Other: hypoxia, pain, constipation, urinary retention, and critical care environment.

Pathophysiology

Delirium results from neurotransmitter imbalances (↓ acetylcholine, ↑ dopamine), neuroinflammation, and oxidative stress. Systemic illness releases pro-inflammatory cytokines (IL-1, IL-6, TNF-α), which cross the blood–brain barrier and interfere with neuronal signalling. Hypoxia and impaired cerebral oxidative metabolism worsen dysfunction, while elevated cortisol and neuroendocrine stress responses add to the effects.

Clinical Features

- Disturbance in attention and awareness
- Acute onset with fluctuating course
- Disorganised thinking and incoherent speech
- Altered consciousness (hyperactive, hypoactive, or mixed)

- Sleep–wake cycle disturbance
- Hallucinations (often visual) or delusions
- Emotional lability or irritability

Subtypes: hyperactive (agitated, hallucinating), hypoactive (withdrawn, easily missed), or mixed.

Management

- Treat the underlying cause (infection, metabolic derangement, drug withdrawal).
- Supportive care: hydration, nutrition, oxygenation, pain relief, and regular toileting.
- Environment: use orientation aids (clocks, calendars, family photos), ensure glasses and hearing aids are available, reduce noise, and promote a normal sleep cycle.
- Medication: antipsychotics (e.g. haloperidol 0.5–1 mg PO/IM) only if severely distressed or unsafe. Avoid benzodiazepines unless treating alcohol/sedative withdrawal.
- Multidisciplinary approach with medical, nursing, pharmacy, and allied health input.

Prognosis

Delirium is associated with higher mortality, extended hospital stays, and long-term cognitive decline. Early detection and treatment improve results, but some patients continue to experience lasting impairment.

Bibliography

Davidson's Principles and Practice of Medicine. 24th ed. Edinburgh: Elsevier; 2022.

Inouye SK. Delirium in older persons. N Engl J Med. 2006;354(11):1157–1165.

Inouye SK, van Dyck LA, Alessi CA, et al. Clarifying confusion: the confusion assessment method (CAM). Ann Intern Med. 1990;113(12):941–948.

Kumar and Clark's Clinical Medicine. 11th ed. Edinburgh: Elsevier; 2023.

MacLullich AMJ, Davis DHJ. Delirium: acute change with long-term implications. Age Ageing. 2018;47(3):323–324.

National Institute for Health and Care Excellence. Delirium: Prevention, Diagnosis and Management (NG103). London: NICE; 2023 https://www.nice.org.uk.

NHS. Delirium. 2024. https://www.nhs.uk.

Oxford Handbook of Clinical Medicine. 11th ed. Oxford: Oxford University Press; 2024.

Scottish Intercollegiate Guidelines Network. Risk Reduction and Management of Delirium (SIGN 157). Edinburgh: SIGN; 2019 https://www.sign.ac.uk.

Wesley Ely E, Inouye SK, Pandharipande PP. Delirium in critically ill patients. Lancet. 2014;383(9920):911–922.

33

Diabetes Mellitus

Diabetes mellitus (DM) is a chronic metabolic disorder characterised by persistent hyperglycaemia caused by insufficient insulin production, impaired insulin action, or both. It is linked to long-term complications affecting the eyes, kidneys, nerves, heart, and blood vessels.

Types

- Type 1 DM (T1DM): autoimmune destruction of pancreatic β-cells results in a complete lack of insulin. It is associated with islet autoantibodies (anti-GAD, IA-2) and typically occurs in childhood or young adulthood, with a rapid onset.
- Type 2 DM (T2DM): the most common form, involving insulin resistance in peripheral tissues with relative insulin deficiency. It is associated with obesity, metabolic syndrome, and chronic low-grade inflammation. Over time, β-cell failure worsens hyperglycaemia.
- Other types: include maturity-onset diabetes of the young (MODY), gestational diabetes, and secondary diabetes (e.g. pancreatitis, steroid-induced).

Pathophysiology

T1DM develops due to autoimmune destruction of pancreatic β-cells. Genetic susceptibility, environmental triggers, and immune dysregulation combine to initiate a process in which autoreactive T lymphocytes target and destroy insulin-producing cells in the islets of Langerhans. Over time, this results in a complete loss of endogenous insulin production. The absence of insulin prevents glucose uptake into peripheral tissues, especially muscle and adipose tissue, leading to uncontrolled hyperglycaemia. Patients with T1DM therefore require lifelong exogenous insulin for survival.

T2DM is more complex and results from a combination of insulin resistance and progressive β-cell dysfunction. In the early stages, dysfunction of adipose tissue plays a key role. Excess fat storage, especially visceral adiposity, promotes the release of free fatty acids into the circulation. These interfere with insulin signalling in muscle and liver, reducing glucose uptake and increasing hepatic gluconeogenesis. Additionally, adipose tissue secretes pro-inflammatory cytokines and exhibits altered adipokine secretion, with decreased adiponectin and increased leptin, further impairing insulin sensitivity. Initially, pancreatic β-cells compensate by increasing insulin secretion, maintaining glucose homeostasis despite resistance. However, chronic metabolic stress eventually causes β-cell exhaustion, apoptosis, and an inability to sustain insulin output. At this stage, relative insulin deficiency develops, and overt diabetes becomes evident.

In both T1DM and T2DM, persistent hyperglycaemia causes tissue damage through various biochemical processes. A key mechanism is the non-enzymatic glycation of proteins, which results in the accumulation of advanced glycation end-products (AGEs). These modify protein structure and function, increase oxidative stress, and trigger inflammatory pathways. AGEs also form cross links with collagen in vessel walls, leading to thickening of basement membranes and reduced vascular elasticity. Over time, these alterations contribute to both microvascular and macrovascular complications. Microvascular damage presents as diabetic retinopathy, nephropathy, and neuropathy, each associated with significant morbidity. Macrovascular issues develop through accelerated atherosclerosis, increasing the risk of coronary artery disease, cerebrovascular disease, and peripheral arterial disease. Therefore, although the initial mechanisms of T1DM and T2DM differ, both conditions ultimately share pathways that cause long-term vascular damage and systemic complications.

Diagnosis

The diagnosis of diabetes is made using specific biochemical criteria, with confirmation typically required through repeat testing in asymptomatic individuals. Several diagnostic pathways are recognised. A fasting plasma glucose level of 7.0 mmol/L or higher indicates diabetes, reflecting impaired basal glucose regulation. Alternatively, a random plasma glucose measurement of 11.1 mmol/L or above, in the presence of typical symptoms such as polyuria, polydipsia, and unexplained weight loss, confirms the diagnosis. Glycated haemoglobin (HbA1c) offers an assessment of average glycaemic control over the previous two to three months, and a value of 48 mmol/mol (6.5%) or higher is diagnostic when measured with a validated assay. Furthermore, the oral glucose tolerance test (OGTT) remains a valuable tool, especially when diagnosis is uncertain; a 2-hour plasma glucose of 11.1 mmol/L or above after ingestion of 75 g of glucose confirms diabetes. These criteria establish a solid framework for diagnosis, enabling early detection and prompt intervention to minimise the risk of long-term complications.

Clinical Features

- Polyuria, polydipsia, weight loss, fatigue, and blurred vision.
- Recurrent infections (e.g. candidiasis, urinary tract infections).
- T2DM may present insidiously or be detected incidentally on screening.

Management

Follow local and national guidelines (e.g. NICE NG17, NG28).

- Lifestyle modification: diet, physical activity, and weight management.
- T1DM: lifelong insulin therapy (basal-bolus or pump).
- T2DM: stepwise approach:
  1) First-line: metformin (if tolerated).
  2) Add-on therapies: sulphonylureas, DPP-4 inhibitors, SGLT2 inhibitors, GLP-1 agonists, or insulin depending on HbA1c, comorbidities, and patient preference.
  3) Optimise cardiovascular risk: statins, antihypertensives, and antiplatelets if indicated.
- Monitoring: HbA1c every 3–6 months, annual screening for complications (retinal screening, urine albumin:creatinine ratio, foot exam).

Diabetic Ketoacidosis (DKA)

A life-threatening acute complication, usually in T1DM.

Pathophysiology

Diabetic ketoacidosis (DKA) occurs when there is an absolute or relative deficiency of insulin, most commonly in type 1 diabetes but occasionally in type 2 diabetes under severe stress conditions. Without sufficient insulin, glucose cannot enter peripheral tissues efficiently, and the body switches to alternative energy sources. Increased lipolysis in adipose tissue releases large amounts of free fatty acids, which are transported to the liver. There, they are converted via β-oxidation into ketone bodies, mainly β-hydroxybutyrate and acetoacetate. The accumulation of these acidic intermediates overwhelms the body's buffering systems, resulting in the high anion gap metabolic acidosis characteristic of DKA.

Hyperglycaemia is a characteristic feature of the condition. Without insulin, hepatic gluconeogenesis and glycogenolysis continue unchecked, resulting in elevated plasma glucose levels. The excess glucose in the bloodstream exceeds the renal threshold for reabsorption, resulting in glycosuria and significant osmotic diuresis. This results in a rapid loss of water and electrolytes, including sodium, potassium, and phosphate, ultimately leading to severe dehydration, volume depletion, and circulatory instability.

The rise in counter-regulatory hormones, such as glucagon, catecholamines, and cortisol, further exacerbates the metabolic disturbances. These hormones enhance gluconeogenesis, glycogenolysis, and lipolysis, sustaining both hyperglycaemia and ketone formation. This cycle of acidosis, dehydration, and electrolyte imbalance hampers tissue perfusion and oxygen delivery, while shifts in potassium between intracellular and extracellular compartments increase the risk of life-threatening arrhythmias. Without prompt recognition and treatment, these processes can quickly lead to shock, cerebral oedema, and multi-organ failure.

Clinical features

- Polyuria, polydipsia, abdominal pain, and vomiting.
- Kussmaul breathing and acetone (fruity) breath.
- Dehydration and hypotension.
- Altered mental status → coma.

Diagnostic criteria (NICE)

- Blood glucose > 11 mmol/L.
- Ketones > 3.0 mmol/L (or ++ on urine dip).
- Venous pH < 7.3 or HCO_3^- < 15 mmol/L.

Management: (trust-specific protocols must be followed)

- ABCDE approach.
- IV fluids (0.9% NaCl for resuscitation).
- Fixed-rate IV insulin infusion (e.g. 0.1 units/kg/hr).
- Potassium replacement guided by serum levels.
- Hourly monitoring of glucose, ketones, VBG, and electrolytes.
- Identify and treat precipitating cause (e.g. infection, missed insulin).

Hyperosmolar Hyperglycaemic State (HHS)

Hyperosmolar hyperglycaemic state (HHS) is a medical emergency, typically observed in older patients with T2DM. It is characterised by severe hyperglycaemia and dehydration without significant ketosis or acidosis.

Pathophysiology: Insulin levels are sufficient to prevent ketogenesis but inadequate to control hyperglycaemia. Severe hyperglycaemia (>30 mmol/L) triggers osmotic diuresis, leading to significant dehydration, electrolyte disturbances, and hyperosmolarity (>320 mOsm/kg). This hyperosmolar state impairs brain function, resulting in confusion, seizures, or coma.

Clinical Features

- Marked hyperglycaemia (often >30 mmol/L).
- Severe dehydration (dry mucous membranes, hypotension, tachycardia).
- Neurological deficits (confusion, seizures, coma).
- Minimal or absent ketones.
- Serum osmolality >320 mOsm/kg.

Management

- ABCDE approach.
- IV fluids: careful and gradual rehydration with 0.9% NaCl.
- Fixed-rate IV insulin (lower dose than DKA, e.g. 0.05 units/kg/hr).

- Potassium replacement as required.
- Monitor osmolality, electrolytes, glucose, and fluid balance.
- Identify and treat precipitating cause (e.g. infection, MI, stroke, medication non-adherence).

Bibliography

American Diabetes Association. Standards of care in diabetes – 2024. Diab Care. 2024;47 (Suppl 1):11–19.

Joint British Diabetes Societies for Inpatient Care (JBDS-IP). Management of hyperosmolar hyperglycaemic state (HHS) in adults. 2023 update.

Kitabchi AE, Umpierrez GE, Miles JM, Fisher JN. Hyperglycemic crises in adult patients with diabetes. Diab Care. 2009;32(7):1335–1343.

National Institute for Health and Care Excellence (NICE). Type 1 diabetes in adults: diagnosis and management (NG17). 2015, updated 2021.

National Institute for Health and Care Excellence (NICE). Type 2 diabetes in adults: management (NG28). 2015, updated 2022.

34

Endocarditis

Infective endocarditis (IE) is a microbial infection of the endocardial surface of the heart, most often affecting valves. It is a life-threatening condition with risks of embolism, sepsis, and heart failure.

Pathophysiology

Endothelial damage (e.g. turbulent flow, prosthetic material) exposes collagen, leading to the formation of platelet–fibrin thrombi (non-bacterial thrombotic endocarditis). When bacteria enter the bloodstream (e.g. through dental work, intravenous drug user [IVDU], or catheters), they adhere to the thrombus via adhesins, forming vegetations composed of fibrin, platelets, and microbes. These are avascular and shielded from host immunity, allowing persistent infection. Vegetations may embolise (→ infarcts, septic emboli) or cause valve destruction and regurgitation.

Common organisms

- Native valves: *Staphylococcus aureus*, *Streptococcus viridans*, and *Enterococcus*
- Prosthetic valves: Coagulase-negative staphylococci and *S. aureus*
- IVDU: *S. aureus* (often tricuspid)
- Culture-negative: Prior antibiotics, or atypicals (Haemophilus, Aggregatibacter, Cardiobacterium, Eikenella and Kingella [HACEK])

Clinical features

- Fever, rigours, and malaise.
- New or changing murmur.
- Embolic signs: stroke, splinter haemorrhages, and Janeway lesions.
- Immunological signs: Osler nodes, Roth spots, and glomerulonephritis.
- Features of heart failure.

Diagnosis (modified Duke criteria)

- Major: typical positive blood cultures; echo indicating vegetation or endocardial involvement.
- Minor: risk factors (e.g. IVDU), fever, vascular or immunological signs, and less-specific microbiology.

Investigations

- 3+ sets of blood cultures (before antibiotics).
- FBC, CRP/ESR, and renal function.
- ECG (conduction block may suggest abscess).
- Echo: TTE (Transthoracic echocardiogram) first; TOE (Transoesophageal echocardiogram) if prosthetic valve or high suspicion.

Management

- Empirical IV antibiotics → tailor to sensitivities; minimum 4–6 weeks.
- Early microbiology input is essential.
- Surgery if: refractory heart failure, abscess, recurrent emboli, or prosthetic valve involvement.
- Monitor for complications (stroke, renal dysfunction).

Prophylaxis

Indicated for selected high-risk patients (prosthetic valves, previous IE) before invasive dental procedures – follow local or national guidance.

Bibliography

Habib G et al. 2015 ESC Guidelines for the management of infective endocarditis. Eur Heart J. 2015;36(44):3075–3128.

National Institute for Health and Care Excellence (NICE). Antimicrobial prophylaxis against infective endocarditis. Clinical guideline CG64. 2016.

35

Ethics in Clinical Practice

Ethics is a fundamental aspect of medicine, influencing how clinicians make decisions, communicate with patients, and interact with society. Unlike clinical guidelines, which offer evidence-based advice, ethics considers what should be done when different values, priorities, or rights conflict. For patients, ethical practice ensures the protection of dignity, autonomy, and trust. For healthcare professionals, it provides a framework for making difficult decisions, particularly when time is limited and the stakes are high.

Ethical challenges are present across all healthcare settings, not just in intensive care or end-of-life scenarios. They occur every day when sharing information, balancing patient autonomy with professional responsibilities, and managing limited resources. Understanding the principles of consent, capacity, end-of-life care, and human factors helps practitioners provide care that is not only safe and effective but also morally appropriate.

Consent and Capacity

Consent underpins all healthcare interventions. In the United Kingdom, the principle is that no patient should receive medical treatment without valid permission unless there is a clear legal or emergency justification. Valid consent must be

- Voluntary: given freely, without coercion.
- Informed: based on an explanation of risks, benefits, and alternatives.
- Given by a person with capacity.

The Mental Capacity Act (2005) sets out the legal framework for assessing capacity in England and Wales. Capacity is specific to each decision and each moment: a person might lack capacity for complex choices but have it for simpler ones, or their capacity may change over time. To lack capacity, an individual must be unable to understand, remember, weigh up, or communicate information relevant to a decision due to an impairment of the mind or brain.

If a patient is found to lack capacity, decisions must be made in their best interests, taking into account their values, beliefs, and previously expressed wishes. This may involve family members, but the final responsibility rests with the healthcare professional. In emergencies, treatment can proceed without consent if it is necessary to preserve life or prevent serious harm, provided it is proportionate and in the patient's best interests.

End-of-Life Decisions

End-of-life care presents some of the most difficult ethical dilemmas in medicine. Choices frequently centre on balancing the extension of life with the provision of comfort and dignity.

Withholding or withdrawing treatment is ethically and legally different from euthanasia. The law recognises that there is no obligation to provide or continue treatment that is futile, burdensome, or against the patient's wishes. A decision not to initiate or discontinue interventions, such as mechanical ventilation or dialysis, is ethically acceptable if it is in the patient's best interests.

Do Not Attempt Cardiopulmonary Resuscitation (DNACPR) orders are a sensitive yet important area. These should be based on clinical judgement, the likelihood of benefit, and the patient's preferences. Whenever possible, discussions should involve the patient and their family openly and compassionately.

Palliative care is essential in end-of-life decision-making. Effective communication, symptom management, and psychological support for both patient and family uphold the principle of dignity at the end of life.

Human Factors and Professionalism

Human factors recognise that healthcare is provided by people working within complex systems, where errors and miscommunication can happen. Ethical practice is therefore not only about individual decisions but also about how teams operate and how organisations support the delivery of safe, compassionate care.

The duty of candour obliges clinicians to be truthful with patients when mistakes happen, providing explanations, apologies, and suitable remedies. These safeguards are based on trust in the patient–clinician relationship.

Teamwork and hierarchy each pose their own ethical challenges. Junior staff might hesitate to raise concerns, or clinicians may encounter 'moral distress' when they feel the appropriate course of action is hindered by organisational constraints. Recognising human factors – communication, leadership, situational awareness, and decision fatigue – is crucial in safeguarding patient safety and supporting staff well-being.

Ethical professionalism also applies to how clinicians care for themselves and one another. Burnout, stress, and moral injury can compromise ethical judgment. Reflection, supervision, and supportive organisational cultures are therefore not luxuries but ethical necessities in maintaining quality care.

Bibliography

Beauchamp TL, Childress JF. Principles of Biomedical Ethics. 8th ed. Oxford: Oxford University Press; 2019.

British Medical Association (BMA). Ethical Guidance for Doctors. London: BMA; 2023.

Department of Health. Mental Capacity Act 2005: Code of Practice. London: The Stationery Office; 2007.

General Medical Council (GMC). Good Medical Practice. London: GMC; 2024.

Nuffield Council on Bioethics. End of Life Care: Ethical Issues. London: Nuffield Council; 2011.

36

The Four Pillars of Advanced Practice

Advanced clinical practice in the United Kingdome is supported by four main pillars: clinical practice, leadership and management, education, and research. Collectively, these areas ensure that advanced practitioners not only provide high-quality care but also contribute to the broader development of healthcare services.

Clinical practice is the foundation of advanced roles. Practitioners demonstrate expert knowledge and skills in complex decision-making, often managing acutely unwell patients or those with multiple comorbidities. This includes advanced assessment, interpretation of investigations, prescribing, and the ability to lead patient management across multidisciplinary teams. The emphasis is on delivering holistic, patient-centred care while working at the boundaries of traditional professional roles.

The second pillar, leadership and management, recognises that advanced practitioners are expected to influence and shape the services in which they work. This may involve leading quality improvement projects, developing clinical pathways, or contributing to workforce planning. Leadership also encompasses supporting colleagues, promoting effective teamwork, and serving as a role model in upholding professional standards. By assuming these responsibilities, advanced practitioners help drive innovation and ensure the delivery of safe and efficient care.

Education is equally important. Advanced practitioners support others' development by teaching, mentoring, and facilitating learning in both formal and informal contexts. They help educate students, junior staff, and colleagues from various professional groups, ensuring that knowledge and skills spread throughout the workforce. Furthermore, advanced practitioners are dedicated to their own ongoing professional development, maintaining their competence and adapting to new evidence and technologies.

The final pillar, research, emphasises the responsibility to advance practice by generating, applying, and sharing evidence. This may involve leading or participating in clinical research, conducting audits and service evaluations, or critically reviewing literature to inform practice. By embedding research into their roles, advanced practitioners ensure care is based on evidence and stays current with the latest developments in healthcare.

Taken together, the four pillars offer a comprehensive framework for advanced practice. They ensure that practitioners not only deliver expert clinical care but also serve as leaders, educators, and innovators who contribute to the ongoing improvement of healthcare systems.

Bibliography

Bryant-Lukosius D, DiCenso A, Browne G, Pinelli J. Advanced practice nursing roles: development, implementation and evaluation. J Adv Nurs. 2004;48(5):519–529.

Department of Health. Modernising Nursing Careers: Advanced Nursing Practice. London: DH; 2006.

Health Education England (HEE). Multi-Professional Framework for Advanced Clinical Practice in England. London: HEE; 2017.

NHS England. Workforce Transformation: Advanced Clinical Practice. London: NHS England; 2022.

Royal College of Nursing (RCN). Advanced Level Nursing: A Position Statement. London: RCN; 2018.

37

Full Blood Count Overview

The full blood count (FBC) is a standard test that provides information about red blood cells, white blood cells (WBCs), and platelets. It is often the initial investigation conducted when evaluating patients in acute and critical care.

Red Blood Cells (RBCs) and Indices

- Haemoglobin (Hb): reflects oxygen-carrying capacity.
- Haematocrit (Hct): proportion of blood volume made up by red blood cells (RBCs).
- Mean corpuscular volume (MCV): RBC size.
  - Microcytic (<80 fL): iron deficiency and thalassaemia
  - Normocytic (80–100 fL): acute blood loss and chronic disease
  - Macrocytic (>100 fL): B12/folate deficiency, alcohol, and marrow disease
- Mean corpuscular haemoglobin (MCH): average Hb per RBC; low in iron deficiency.
- Red cell distribution width (RDW): variation in cell size; high in mixed anaemias.

White Blood Cells (WBCs)

- Total white cell count (WCC) raised in infection, inflammation, and steroids; low in sepsis, viral infections, and marrow suppression.
- Neutrophils: bacterial infection, stress, and steroids.
- Lymphocytes: viral infections and chronic lymphotcytic leukemia (CLL) reduced in stress or immunosuppression.
- Monocytes: chronic infection (e.g. TB, endocarditis).
- Eosinophils: allergy and parasites.
- Basophils: hypersensitivity and myeloproliferative disease.

Platelets

- Count:
  - Low (thrombocytopenia): sepsis, DIC, marrow failure, and drugs.
  - High (thrombocytosis): inflammation, iron deficiency, and malignancy.
- Mean platelet volume (MPV): larger platelets suggest increased turnover.

Bibliography

British Society for Haematology. *Guidelines and Resources for Haematological Investigations.* London: BSH; 2022 https://b-s-h.org.uk.

Dacie and Lewis Practical Haematology. 13th ed. Philadelphia: Elsevier; 2021.

Davidson's Principles and Practice of Medicine. 24th ed. Edinburgh: Elsevier; 2022.

Hoffbrand's Essential Haematology. 8th ed. Hoboken: Wiley-Blackwell; 2023.

Kumar and Clark's Clinical Medicine. 11th ed. Edinburgh: Elsevier; 2023.

National Institute for Health and Care Excellence. Blood Tests – Full Blood Count. London: NICE; 2023 https://www.nice.org.uk.

NHS. Full blood count (FBC). 2024. https://www.nhs.uk

Oxford Handbook of Clinical Haematology. 5th ed. Oxford: Oxford University Press; 2023.

Royal College of Pathologists. *Guidelines on the Interpretation of Laboratory Blood Tests.* London: RCPath; 2021 https://www.rcpath.org.

38

Gastrointestinal Bleeding

Gastrointestinal bleeding refers to blood loss originating from any part of the gastrointestinal tract. It is generally classified as either upper or lower, depending on whether the source is proximal or distal to the ligament of Treitz. Peptic ulcer disease, oesophageal varices, Mallory–Weiss tears, or erosive gastritis are the most common causes of upper GI bleeds. Conversely, lower GI bleeds are often caused by diverticular disease, colorectal cancer, angiodysplasia, or inflammatory bowel disease. The clinical presentation varies widely: haematemesis and melaena are typical signs of upper GI bleeding, while haematochezia is more common with lower GI bleeding; however, brisk upper bleeds can present with fresh rectal blood if the transit time is rapid.

Pathophysiology

The underlying mechanisms of GI bleeding reflect the balance between mucosal defences, vascular integrity, and haemodynamic responses. In peptic ulcer disease, chronic exposure to gastric acid and pepsin disrupts mucosal defences, allowing erosion into the underlying vasculature. Once arterial vessels are breached, haemorrhage may be brisk and life-threatening. In variceal bleeding, portal hypertension arising from cirrhosis or other causes forces blood into collateral venous pathways, producing fragile, dilated varices within the oesophagus or stomach. These thin-walled vessels rupture easily under increased pressure, leading to massive haemorrhage.

Mallory–Weiss tears occur due to sudden increases in intra-abdominal pressure, such as severe vomiting, leading to mucosal lacerations at the gastro-oesophageal junction. Lower GI sources differ in their mechanism: diverticulosis results in outpouchings of the colonic wall where penetrating vessels are stretched and may erode, while angiodysplasia involves dilated, thin-walled mucosal vessels that are prone to bleeding under minimal stress.

Regardless of the cause, significant bleeding decreases circulating volume and impairs tissue perfusion. The body initially compensates through sympathetic activation, tachycardia, and peripheral vasoconstriction. If blood loss continues, hypovolaemic shock occurs, affecting oxygen delivery to vital organs. Lactic acidosis and anaerobic metabolism then ensue, worsening cellular injury. In variceal bleeds, systemic effects are further exacerbated by coagulopathy, infection risk, and diminished hepatic reserve, all of which heighten morbidity and mortality.

Assessment

A structured ABCDE approach should guide the initial assessment. The airway must be secured, particularly in patients with ongoing haematemesis or reduced consciousness. Oxygen is administered to optimise tissue delivery, and circulation is rapidly addressed with two large-bore IV cannulas, isotonic fluids, and early activation of the primary haemorrhage protocol when necessary. Transfusion should balance red blood cells with plasma and platelets, typically in a 1:1:1 ratio for massive bleeds. Clinical markers of shock – such as tachycardia, hypotension, cold extremities, and altered mental status – should be closely monitored.

Investigations

Key investigations include

- Bedside: capillary glucose and arterial/venous blood gas to assess lactate and acid–base status.
- Laboratory: FBC, U&Es, LFTs, clotting screen, group and save, and crossmatch.
- Imaging: CXR if aspiration or perforation is suspected; CT angiography or tagged red cell scanning for persistent but unlocalised bleeding.
- Risk stratification: tools like the Glasgow–Blatchford Score (GBS) and Rockall Score assist in assessing the urgency of endoscopy and the required level of care (Blatchford et al., 2000; Rockall et al., 1996).

Pharmacological Management

Medical therapy is initiated alongside resuscitation. Intravenous proton pump inhibitors (e.g. omeprazole 80 mg bolus followed by an 8 mg/hr infusion) reduce gastric acid secretion and stabilise clot formation in suspected peptic ulcer disease. In suspected variceal haemorrhage, terlipressin decreases portal pressure, while prophylactic antibiotics such as ceftriaxone lower the risk of infection and enhance survival. Anticoagulation should be reversed promptly where appropriate, using vitamin K, prothrombin complex concentrate, or specific antidotes.

Definitive Management

Definitive treatment is usually endoscopic. Upper GI endoscopy should be performed within 24 hours once the patient is stabilised, providing both diagnosis and therapy options, including adrenaline injection, thermal coagulation, haemostatic clips, or band ligation of varices. Colonoscopy is preferred for lower GI bleeds after appropriate resuscitation and bowel preparation. Interventional radiology (e.g. embolisation) may be required for refractory or anatomically challenging cases, while surgery remains a last resort for uncontrolled haemorrhage or complications such as perforation.

Bibliography

Blatchford O, Murray WR, Blatchford M. A risk score to predict need for treatment for upper-gastrointestinal haemorrhage. Lancet. 2000;356(9238):1318–1321.

British Society of Gastroenterology (BSG). Guidelines on the management of acute lower gastrointestinal bleeding. 2019.

Laine L, Jensen DM. Management of patients with ulcer bleeding. Am J Gastroenterol. 2012;107(3):345–360.

National Institute for Health and Care Excellence (NICE). Acute upper gastrointestinal bleeding in over 16s: management (CG141). 2016.

Resuscitation Council UK. Advanced life support guidelines. 2021.

Rockall TA, Logan RF, Devlin HB, Northfield TC. Risk assessment after acute upper gastrointestinal haemorrhage. Gut. 1996;38(3):316–321.

Strate LL, Gralnek IM. Management of patients with acute lower gastrointestinal bleeding. N Engl J Med. 2016;374(8):787–789.

Tripathi D, Stanley AJ, Hayes PC, et al. UK guidelines on the management of variceal haemorrhage in cirrhotic patients. Gut. 2015;64(11):1680–1704.

Villanueva C, Colomo A, Bosch A, et al. Transfusion strategies for acute upper gastrointestinal bleeding. N Engl J Med. 2014;368(1):11–21.

39

Guillain–Barré Syndrome

Guillain–Barré syndrome (GBS) is an acute, immune-mediated polyneuropathy typically triggered by infection, characterised by rapidly progressing, symmetrical weakness with diminished or absent reflexes. Weakness usually starts in the lower limbs and ascends.

Pathophysiology

GBS results from molecular mimicry, where antibodies produced against pathogens cross-react with components of the peripheral nervous system. The most common trigger is *Campylobacter jejuni*, although viruses like CMV, EBV, influenza, *Mycoplasma pneumoniae*, and SARS-CoV-2 are also involved. In acute inflammatory demyelinating polyradiculoneuropathy (AIDP), macrophages and T cells attack myelin, disrupting saltatory conduction and leading to weakness. In axonal variants (e.g. acute motor axonal neuropathy [AMAN]), antibodies target gangliosides on motor axons, causing rapid paralysis. Autonomic fibres may also be affected, resulting in arrhythmias and blood pressure instability.

Clinical Features

- Symmetrical, progressive limb weakness (ascending pattern).
- Areflexia or hyporeflexia.
- Sensory symptoms (paraesthesia, numbness).
- Cranial/bulbar involvement: dysphagia and facial weakness.
- Autonomic dysfunction: BP lability, arrhythmias, and urinary retention.
- Respiratory failure in severe cases.

Variants include AIDP (most common in Europe), AMAN (prevalent in Asia and Latin America), and Miller Fisher syndrome (characterised by ophthalmoplegia, ataxia, and areflexia).

Diagnosis

GBS is mainly diagnosed clinically, but is supported by

- Nerve conduction studies/EMG indicating demyelination or axonal loss.
- CSF → albuminocytologic dissociation (elevated protein, normal WCC).
- Antiganglioside antibodies (e.g. GM1, GQ1b) in variants.

Management

- IV immunoglobulin (IVIG) or plasma exchange – equally effective when initiated early.
- Supportive care: monitor vital capacity, cardiac rhythm, and fluid balance; provide thromboprophylaxis and nutrition.
- Rehabilitation: physiotherapy and occupational therapy.

Prognosis

- 80% recover completely or nearly completely.
- 5–10% with long-term disability.
- Mortality rate of 2–5%, usually caused by respiratory or autonomic complications.

Bibliography

Hughes RAC, Cornblath DR. Guillain-Barré syndrome. Lancet. 2005;366(9497):1653–1666.

Sejvar JJ et al. Population incidence of Guillain-Barré syndrome: a systematic review and meta-analysis. Neuroepidemiology. 2011;36(2):123–133.

Willison HJ, Jacobs BC, van Doorn PA. Guillain-Barré syndrome. Lancet. 2016;388(10045):717–727.

40

Haematological Cancers and Emergencies

Haematological cancers affect the blood, bone marrow, and lymphatic system, resulting from the uncontrolled growth of abnormal blood cells or their precursors. They may present with either slowly developing symptoms or acute emergencies requiring immediate intervention.

Major Haematological Malignancies

- Acute lymphoblastic leukaemia (ALL): malignant proliferation of lymphoblasts, most common in children, presenting with marrow failure and rapid progression.
- Acute myeloid leukaemia (AML): clonal proliferation of myeloid blasts, frequently associated with pancytopenia and an aggressive progression.
- Chronic lymphocytic leukaemia (CLL): gradual build-up of dysfunctional B lymphocytes; often asymptomatic with incidental lymphocytosis.
- Chronic myeloid leukaemia (CML): caused by the BCR–ABL fusion gene (Philadelphia chromosome), resulting in unchecked tyrosine kinase activity.
- Hodgkin lymphoma (HL): characterised by Reed–Sternberg cells, usually presenting with localised lymphadenopathy and systemic 'B' symptoms.
- Non-Hodgkin lymphoma (NHL): a diverse group with varying progression, from slow-growing to highly aggressive.
- Multiple myeloma: malignant proliferation of plasma cells, leading to lytic bone lesions, marrow failure, renal dysfunction, and abnormal immunoglobulin production.

General Management

Diagnosis involves blood tests, a bone marrow biopsy, and imaging. Treatment includes chemotherapy, immunotherapy (e.g. monoclonal antibodies), targeted therapies (e.g. tyrosine kinase inhibitors in CML), radiotherapy, and stem cell transplantation. Supportive measures such as transfusions, infection prevention, and bisphosphonates for bone disease are essential.

Haematological Emergencies

Certain acute complications may be the initial presentation of malignancy or occur during treatment.

- Tumour lysis syndrome (TLS): rapid cell destruction releases uric acid, potassium, and phosphate, leading to renal injury, hyperkalaemia, and hypocalcaemia. Common after chemotherapy for acute leukaemias or high-grade lymphomas. Management involves IV hydration, rasburicase or allopurinol, electrolyte monitoring, and dialysis if severe.
- Disseminated intravascular coagulation (DIC): systemic activation of coagulation causes microthrombosis, consumes clotting factors, and leads to bleeding. Causes include sepsis, trauma, obstetric complications, and malignancy. Labs show low platelets, prolonged PT/aPTT, low fibrinogen, and raised D-dimer. Management involves treating the underlying cause, providing supportive transfusions (fresh frozen plasma [FFP] cryoprecipitate, platelets), and carefully balancing anticoagulation.
- Thrombotic thrombocytopenic purpura (TTP): caused by ADAMTS13 deficiency leading to large von Willebrand Facotr (vWF) multimers, which promote platelet aggregation and microvascular thrombosis. Features include thrombocytopenia, haemolytic anaemia, renal impairment, neurological signs, and fever. It is a medical emergency requiring plasma exchange and steroids.
- Acute anaemia/haemolysis: a rapid decline in haemoglobin levels may result from bleeding, haemolysis (e.g. autoimmune, G6PD deficiency), or marrow failure; treated with transfusion, oxygen, and disease-specific therapy (e.g. steroids for autoimmune haemolysis).
- Heparin-induced thrombocytopenia (HIT): an immune-mediated prothrombotic disorder that occurs 5–10 days after heparin exposure. It is caused by antibodies against platelet factor 4-heparin complexes, leading to thrombosis despite low platelet counts. Management involves discontinuing heparin and initiating a non-heparin anticoagulant.

Bibliography

Connors JM. Hodgkin lymphoma: treatment. N Engl J Med. 2017;378:446–460.

Döhner H, Weisdorf DJ, Bloomfield CD. Acute myeloid leukemia. N Engl J Med. 2015;373:1136–1152.

George JN. Thrombotic thrombocytopenic purpura. N Engl J Med. 2006;354:1927–1935.

Hallek M et al. Chronic lymphocytic leukaemia: ESMO Clinical Practice Guidelines. Ann Oncol. 2018;29(Suppl 4):iv192–iv199.

Hochhaus A et al. Chronic myeloid leukaemia: ESMO Clinical Practice Guidelines. Ann Oncol. 2017;28(Suppl 4):iv41–iv51.

Howard SC et al. Tumor lysis syndrome in children with malignancies. N Engl J Med. 2011;364:1844–1854.

Levi M, Ten Cate H. Disseminated intravascular coagulation. N Engl J Med. 1999;341:586–592.
Swerdlow SH, Campo E, Harris NL, et al. WHO Classification of Tumours of Haematopoietic and Lymphoid Tissues. IARC; 2017.
Warkentin TE. Heparin-induced thrombocytopenia: pathogenesis and management. Br J Haematol. 2003;121:535–555.

41

Heart Failure

Heart failure is a clinical syndrome where the heart cannot pump enough blood to meet metabolic needs. It may result from impaired ventricular filling or decreased ejection, usually due to ischaemic heart disease, hypertension, or valvular problems.

Classification

Type	Definition	Key Causes
HFrEF	EF $< 40\%$	MI, dilated cardiomyopathy
HFpEF	EF $\geq 50\%$	Hypertension, ageing, and obesity
Acute versus chronic	Sudden versus gradual onset	MI and arrhythmia (acute); valve disease and HTN (chronic)
Left versus right	Pulmonary versus systemic congestion	Often coexist

Clinical Features

- Left-sided failure: dyspnoea, orthopnoea, paroxysmal nocturnal dyspnoea (PND), pulmonary crackles, pink frothy sputum, and fatigue.
- Right-sided failure: peripheral oedema, ascites, hepatomegaly, raised JVP, and weight gain.

Causes (Mnemonic: FAILURE)

- F: Faulty valves
- A: Arrhythmias
- I: Infarction (MI)
- L: Lineage (genetics)

- U: Uncontrolled hypertension
- R: Recreational drugs/toxins
- E: Endocrine (thyroid, diabetes)

Pathophysiology

Heart failure begins with a decrease in cardiac output, triggering neurohormonal activation. The sympathetic nervous system (SNS) raises heart rate and contractility, while the renin–angiotensin–aldosterone system (RAAS) causes vasoconstriction, as well as sodium and water retention. Although initially compensatory, these mechanisms increase preload and afterload, elevate myocardial oxygen demand, and contribute to maladaptive ventricular remodelling.

- In left-sided failure, pulmonary venous pressures increase, causing pulmonary oedema, impaired gas exchange, and dyspnoea.
- In right-sided failure, systemic venous congestion occurs, leading to hepatomegaly, ascites, and peripheral oedema.
  Persistent neurohormonal activation sustains a vicious cycle of worsening dysfunction and clinical decompensation.

Investigations

- BNP/NT-proBNP: elevated in HF (low values exclude diagnosis).
- ECG: ischaemia, arrhythmias, and Left Ventricular Hypertrophy (LVH).
- CXR: cardiomegaly and pulmonary oedema.
- Echocardiography: ejection fraction, wall motion, and valvular disease.
- Bloods: U&Es, FBC, LFTs, and troponin.

Management

Acute

- High-flow O_2, IV furosemide, GTN, and morphine (for selected patients).
- Non-invasive ventilation in cases of respiratory failure.
- Address reversible causes (e.g. MI, arrhythmia).

Chronic (stepwise)

- ACE inhibitor (or ARNI) combined with β-blocker.
- Add mineralocorticoid receptor antagonist (spironolactone).
- Consider SGLT2 inhibitors, ivabradine, and hydralazine/isosorbide in selected groups.
- Device therapy (ICD, CRT) for refractory disease.
- Lifestyle: salt restriction, fluid management, daily weights, and exercise programmes.

Complications

- Pulmonary oedema
- Arrhythmias (AF, VT)
- Cardiorenal or cardiohepatic syndrome
- Thromboembolism
- Sudden cardiac death

Bibliography

British Society for Heart Failure. Clinical Guidance and Resources for Heart Failure Management. London: BSHF; 2022 https://www.bsh.org.uk.

European Society of Cardiology. ESC guidelines for the diagnosis and treatment of acute and chronic heart failure. Eur Heart J. 2021;42(36):3599–3726.

National Institute for Health and Care Excellence (2018, updated 2023) Chronic Heart Failure in Adults: Diagnosis and Management (NG106). London: NICE. https://www.nice.org.uk

National Institute for Health and Care Excellence. Acute Heart Failure: Diagnosis and Management (CG187). London: NICE; 2020 https://www.nice.org.uk.

NHS. Heart failure. 2024. https://www.nhs.uk

Packer M, McMurray JJV. Importance of neurohormonal pathways in heart failure. The Lancet. 2021;398(10304):103–115.

42

Hepatitis

Hepatitis is an inflammation of the liver, typically caused by viral infections, but also by alcohol, certain drugs, autoimmune diseases, and metabolic conditions. It can occur suddenly or develop into a chronic disease, depending on the cause and the body's response. Chronic hepatitis poses a significant risk of cirrhosis, portal hypertension, and hepatocellular carcinoma (HCC).

Pathophysiology

The liver's key functions in detoxification, protein synthesis, and bile production make it susceptible to injury. Hepatitis occurs when hepatocytes are damaged by direct cytotoxic effects, such as those caused by alcohol, drugs, viruses, or the host's immune response. For example, viral hepatitis involves cytotoxic T lymphocytes targeting infected hepatocytes, which leads to necrosis and apoptosis. This immune-mediated damage causes liver cell swelling, lobular inflammation, and, in chronic cases, progressive fibrosis. Activated stellate cells deposit extracellular matrix, which distorts the liver's structure and creates regenerative nodules – signs of cirrhosis. Ongoing injury, especially from hepatitis B or C, establishes a pro-oncogenic environment that increases the risk of HCC.

Types and Key Features

Type	Transmission	Acute/Chronic	Notes
A (HAV)	Faeco-oral	Acute only	Self-limiting; often travel-related
B (HBV)	Blood, sex, and vertical	Both	Vaccine available; ↑ risk of cirrhosis/HCC
C (HCV)	Blood (intravenous drug user) transfusions	Chronic	Often silent until advanced; curable with direct acting antiviralss
D (HDV)	Requires HBV	Chronic	Severe co-infection or superinfection
E (HEV)	Faeco-oral	Acute (except in immunocompromised)	Severe in pregnancy (esp. 3rd trimester)

Clinical Features

- Acute hepatitis: fever, malaise, anorexia, nausea, right upper quadrant pain, jaundice, and hepatomegaly.
- Chronic hepatitis: often asymptomatic until complications like cirrhosis or portal hypertension develop.
- Extra-hepatic features: rash, arthralgia (HBV), cryoglobulinemia, or glomerulonephritis (HCV).

Investigations

- LFTs: hepatocellular pattern (↑ ALT/AST).
- Viral serology: defines type and chronicity.
- Coagulation profile: prolonged INR indicates impaired synthetic function.
- Ultrasound of the liver: evaluates parenchyma and vasculature.
- Fibroscan or biopsy: used for staging fibrosis in chronic cases.

Management

- Acute hepatitis: mainly supportive care (hydration, rest, avoid alcohol and hepatotoxins).
- Antiviral therapy
  - HBV: nucleos(t)ide analogues (e.g. tenofovir, entecavir).
  - HCV: direct-acting antivirals (e.g. sofosbuvir, ledipasvir).
- Prevention
  - Vaccines (HAV, HBV).
  - Safe sex, needle exchange, and screened blood products.
- Public health: notifiable infections (A, B, C, E).

Complications

- Fulminant hepatic failure (rare, acute).
- Chronic hepatitis advancing to cirrhosis and portal hypertension.
- Hepatocellular carcinoma (especially with HBV and HCV).
- Co-infection (e.g. HBV + HDV) hastens disease progression.

Bibliography

European Association for the Study of the Liver (EASL). Clinical practice guidelines: hepatitis B, C, and E. J Hepatol. 2017–2020;83.

NICE. Hepatitis B and C Testing: People at Risk of Infection. NG183. Public Health Guidance; 2020.

World Health Organization. Hepatitis Fact Sheets. WHO; 2023.

43

Hypertension

Hypertension, or high blood pressure, is a chronic condition characterised by persistently elevated arterial pressure. It is a significant risk factor for cardiovascular disease, stroke, renal failure, and aortic aneurysm. The condition is usually asymptomatic and is most often detected during routine monitoring. According to NICE and ESC/ESH guidelines, the diagnostic threshold is a clinic blood pressure of 140/90 mmHg or higher, or an average ambulatory or home blood pressure of 135/85 mmHg or higher.

Classification

Blood pressure is classified by severity, considering both systolic and diastolic readings.

- Normal: <120/<80 mmHg.
- Elevated (high-normal): 120–139/80–89 mmHg.
- Stage 1 hypertension: 140–159/90–99 mmHg.
- Stage 2 hypertension: ≥160/≥100 mmHg.
- Severe hypertension: ≥180/≥120 mmHg.

Causes

Most cases (90–95%) are primary or essential hypertension, where no single cause is identified. Instead, it arises from a combination of genetic susceptibility and lifestyle factors such as obesity, high salt consumption, physical inactivity, excessive alcohol intake, and smoking.

The remaining 5–10% of cases are secondary hypertension, caused by an underlying condition. Common causes include renal disease (e.g. glomerulonephritis, polycystic kidney disease); endocrine disorders such as primary hyperaldosteronism, phaeochromocytoma, and Cushing's syndrome; vascular conditions like renal artery stenosis or coarctation of the aorta; and certain drugs, including NSAIDs, corticosteroids, oral contraceptives, and recreational substances such as cocaine. Obstructive sleep apnoea is also a recognised secondary cause.

Pathophysiology

The interaction between cardiac output and systemic vascular resistance determines blood pressure. In hypertension, this balance is disrupted by several mechanisms. Increased sympathetic nervous system activity and overactivation of the renin–angiotensin–aldosterone system (RAAS) contribute to vasoconstriction and sodium retention. Endothelial dysfunction decreases nitric oxide availability, impairing vasodilatation, while vascular remodelling and increased peripheral resistance further raise pressure. Impaired renal sodium handling (natriuresis) promotes volume expansion, worsening the rise in blood pressure.

Sustained hypertension damages arterial walls, leading to arteriosclerosis, decreased vascular compliance, and end-organ damage. The most affected systems are the heart, where left ventricular hypertrophy occurs; the kidneys, where nephrosclerosis contributes to chronic kidney disease; the brain, with increased risk of stroke and transient ischaemic attack; and the retina, where hypertensive retinopathy can result in vision loss.

Clinical Features

Hypertension is often called the 'silent killer' because most patients are asymptomatic until complications occur. When symptoms are present, they may include morning headaches, dizziness, or blurred vision. Evidence of end-organ damage may be identified through examination or investigations, such as left ventricular hypertrophy, proteinuria, retinal changes (including cotton-wool spots, flame haemorrhages, or papilloedema), and neurological events (such as stroke or transient ischaemic attack).

Investigations

Assessment begins with an accurate blood pressure measurement, ideally using ambulatory blood pressure monitoring (ABPM) or home monitoring to confirm persistent elevation. Additional investigations aim to identify secondary causes, assess cardiovascular risk, and evaluate end-organ damage. These include urinalysis for proteinuria or haematuria, renal function tests (U&Es, creatinine, eGFR), fasting glucose and lipid profile, and an ECG to detect left ventricular hypertrophy or ischaemia. Fundoscopy may reveal retinal changes, while specific tests, such as the plasma aldosterone/renin ratio or urinary catecholamines, are performed if secondary hypertension is suspected.

Management

Management of hypertension involves a gradual pharmacological strategy as described in NICE guidelines.

- Step 1: Patients under 55 years old, or not of Black African or Caribbean heritage, are typically started on an ACE inhibitor such as ramipril. Those over 55 or of Black ethnicity are offered a calcium channel blocker like amlodipine.
- Step 2: Combination therapy with an ACE inhibitor (or ARB) and a calcium channel blocker.
- Step 3: Addition of a thiazide-like diuretic such as indapamide.
- Step 4: If blood pressure remains uncontrolled, consider adding spironolactone if potassium levels allow, or an alpha- or beta-blocker as alternatives.

Lifestyle interventions, such as weight loss, reducing salt intake, increasing physical activity, moderating alcohol consumption, and quitting smoking, remain vital throughout.

Complications

The complications of sustained hypertension are extensive and contribute to significant morbidity and mortality. Cardiovascular issues include left ventricular hypertrophy, heart failure, and myocardial infarction. Cerebrovascular effects encompass stroke, transient ischaemic attack, and vascular dementia. Renal problems involve chronic kidney disease and progressive nephrosclerosis. Vascular complications such as peripheral arterial disease and aortic dissection can occur, along with ophthalmic issues like hypertensive retinopathy and vision loss.

Bibliography

National Institute for Health and Care Excellence (NICE). Hypertension in Adults: Diagnosis and Management (NG136). NICE; 2019 (updated 2023).

National Institute for Health and Care Excellence (NICE). Chronic Kidney Disease: Assessment and Management (NG203). NICE; 2021.

Public Health England. UK Hypertension Guidelines and Blood Pressure Targets. PHE; 2020.

Williams B, Mancia G, Spiering W, et al. 2018 ESC/ESH Guidelines for the management of arterial hypertension. Eur Heart J. 2018;39(33):3021–3104.

44

Intercostal Chest Drains

Intercostal chest drains (ICDs), also known as chest tubes, are used to evacuate air, blood, pus, or other fluids from the pleural space, thereby restoring normal intrapleural pressure and facilitating lung re-expansion.

Indications

Common indications include pneumothorax (spontaneous, traumatic, or tension), haemothorax, pleural effusion (malignant, infective, or inflammatory), empyema, chylothorax, and post-operative drainage following thoracic surgery.

Insertion

Chest drains are inserted using aseptic technique, with analgesia or local anaesthetic, and complete monitoring. The recommended insertion site is the safe triangle, bordered by the anterior edge of latissimus dorsi, the lateral edge of pectoralis major, and a line just above the nipple (5th intercostal space) (BTS, 2010). Ultrasound guidance is recommended for effusions. Once inserted, the drain is attached to an underwater seal or suction, and its position is confirmed by chest X-ray.

Monitoring and Management

Function is evaluated by observing respiration (patency), bubbling during expiration (indicating an air leak), and recording the output volume and character. Patient monitoring should include observations such as respiratory rate, oxygen saturation, and haemodynamic status, as well as repeat imaging. Suction, typically from −10 to −20 cmH_2O, may be necessary for persistent pneumothorax or poorly draining effusions.

Troubleshooting

- Absent swinging: tube blockage, kinking, or malposition.
- Continuous bubbling: persistent air leak, such as bronchopleural fistula.
- Sudden blockage in drainage: clot, kinking, or dislodgement.

Complications

Insertion carries risks such as malposition, infection, haemorrhage, visceral injury (lung, liver, spleen), and re-expansion pulmonary oedema if fluid is removed too rapidly.

Removal

A drain can be removed when the underlying pathology has resolved, drainage is less than 200 mL/24 hours (for fluid), and there is no ongoing air leak. Removal is performed during expiration or a Valsalva manoeuvre, with an immediate occlusive dressing applied. Follow-up imaging confirms resolution.

Bibliography

Havelock T, Teoh R, Laws D, Gleeson F, BTS Pleural Disease Guideline Group. Pleural procedures and thoracic ultrasound: British Thoracic Society Pleural Disease Guideline 2010. Thorax. 2010;65(Suppl 2):ii61–ii76.

Roberts DJ, Leigh-Smith S, Faris PD, et al. Clinical presentation of patients with tension pneumothorax: a systematic review. Ann Surg. 2015;261(6):1068–1078.

45

Heart Sounds

Heart sounds originate from the closure of valves and the movement of blood through the heart during the cardiac cycle.

- Normal sounds
  - S1 (lub): mitral and tricuspid closure, best heard at the apex.
  - S2 (dub): aortic/pulmonary closure, best heard at the base. Physiological splitting during inspiration is normal; wide or fixed splitting indicates atrial septal defects (ASD), while paradoxical splitting suggests left bundle branch block (LBBB) or aortic stenosis (AS).
- Additional sounds
  - S3: early diastole and ventricular gallop; normal in young and pathological in HF.
  - S4: late diastole and atrial gallop; caused by stiff ventricle (e.g. LVH, HTN).
- Murmurs: turbulent flow. Classified by timing (systolic/diastolic), shape, location, radiation, pitch/quality, and response to manoeuvres.
  - Aortic stenosis: harsh systolic ejection murmur, radiates to carotids.
  - Mitral regurgitation: pansystolic, radiates to the axilla.
  - Aortic regurgitation: early diastolic decrescendo, sitting forward.
  - Mitral stenosis: mid-diastolic rumbling, with an opening snap.

Bibliography

McGee S. Evidence-Based Physical Diagnosis. 5th ed. Elsevier; 2021.

NICE. Chronic heart failure in adults: diagnosis and management [NG106]. 2018.

The British Society of Echocardiography. Clinical indications for echocardiography. 2019.

46

Lifelong Learning and Reflective Practice

Healthcare is an ever-changing field. New evidence, technologies, and treatment methods regularly emerge, and what was once considered best practice can quickly become outdated. For healthcare professionals, this reality makes lifelong learning not just desirable but vital. Alongside acquiring new knowledge and skills, reflective practice offers a framework for self-awareness and ongoing improvement, ensuring that clinical decisions remain both evidence-based and patient-centred.

Lifelong learning involves the continuous, voluntary pursuit of knowledge and development throughout a professional career. In healthcare, this encompasses formal education, such as postgraduate courses and specialist training, as well as informal activities, including reading journals, participating in clinical discussions, and on-the-job learning.

Continuing professional development (CPD) is a mandatory requirement for many professions. Organisations such as the General Medical Council (GMC), Nursing and Midwifery Council (NMC), and Health and Care Professions Council (HCPC) mandate that clinicians regularly update and record their CPD to stay on the professional register. Beyond these regulatory frameworks, lifelong learning is crucial for maintaining safe practice, enhancing professional credibility, and adapting to a rapidly evolving healthcare environment.

Modern healthcare increasingly emphasises evidence-based practice, requiring clinicians to evaluate research and incorporate it into clinical decisions critically. Skills such as literature searching, guideline appraisal, and data interpretation are therefore essential for lifelong learning. Equally vital is learning from patients and colleagues, valuing the insights gained through shared experiences and collaborative practice.

Reflective Practice

Reflection is the process of analysing experiences to learn from them and improve future practice. It involves stepping back from an event, considering what went well, what could have been done differently, and how similar situations might be managed in the future. Reflection transforms experience into learning, linking theory with practice.

Several models exist to guide reflective practice, including Gibbs' Reflective Cycle and Schön's concepts of reflection-in-action and reflection-on-action. These frameworks encourage clinicians to move beyond simple description and toward critical analysis, helping them identify underlying assumptions, emotions, and areas for growth. Reflective writing, supervision, and debriefing are practical tools that promote this process.

Benefits of Reflection

Reflective practice offers numerous benefits. For individuals, it enhances clinical judgement, boosts self-awareness, and encourages professional development. By recognising strengths and weaknesses, clinicians can focus on areas needing improvement and increase confidence in their skills. Reflection also supports emotional health, helping practitioners process difficult experiences and lowering the risk of moral distress or burnout.

At a team and organisational level, reflective practice fosters learning cultures where openness and ongoing improvement are valued. Sharing reflections during teaching sessions, at morbidity and mortality meetings, or after critical incidents encourages collective learning and helps prevent the recurrence of errors.

Linking Lifelong Learning and Reflection

Lifelong learning and reflective practice are deeply interconnected. Reflection identifies learning needs, which then inform CPD activities. Conversely, lifelong learning supplies new knowledge and frameworks that can be applied and assessed through reflection. Together, they create a cycle of development where experiences shape learning, and learning influences future practice. This ongoing process ensures that care remains adaptable, evidence-based, and attuned to patients' needs.

Challenges and Barriers

Despite their importance, lifelong learning and reflective practice face challenges. Time pressures, heavy workloads, and organisational cultures that prioritise productivity over development can restrict opportunities for meaningful learning. Some clinicians may view reflection as a bureaucratic exercise required for appraisal or revalidation, rather than a genuine tool for personal growth. Overcoming these obstacles requires strong leadership, protected time for CPD, and creating environments where learning and reflection are valued as essential for safe, high-quality care.

Bibliography

General Medical Council (GMC). Guidance on Reflection and Reflective Practice. London: GMC; 2018.

Gibbs G. Learning by Doing: A Guide to Teaching and Learning Methods. Oxford: Oxford Further Education Unit; 1988.

Kolb DA. Experiential Learning: Experience as the Source of Learning and Development. 2nd ed. New Jersey: Pearson Education; 2014.

Nursing and Midwifery Council (NMC). Realising Professionalism: Standards for Education and Training – Part 1. London: NMC; 2018.

Schön DA. The Reflective Practitioner: How Professionals Think in Action. New York: Basic Books; 1983.

47

Liver Failure and Liver Function Tests

Liver failure is a potentially fatal condition where the liver cannot perform its synthetic, metabolic, and detoxification functions. It may present as

- Acute liver failure – rapid deterioration of a previously healthy liver (e.g. paracetamol overdose, viral hepatitis).
- Chronic liver failure – progressive decompensation caused by cirrhosis (e.g. alcohol, viral hepatitis, non-alcoholic fatty liver disease [NAFLD]).
- Acute-on-chronic liver failure (ACLF) – an acute insult superimposed on chronic disease, often resulting in multi-organ failure.

Pathophysiology

Liver failure occurs when extensive hepatocyte damage exceeds the liver's ability to perform its metabolic, synthetic, and detoxifying roles. This can happen suddenly, as in acute liver failure, or develop gradually in chronic liver disease, leading to decompensation. Regardless of the cause, the inability of hepatocellular functions disrupts homeostasis across various systems.

One of the most notable effects is the build-up of nitrogenous waste products, especially ammonia. In healthy individuals, ammonia is processed through the urea cycle and safely excreted. However, in liver failure, impaired detoxification causes ammonia to accumulate in the circulation, cross the blood–brain barrier, and affect astrocyte function by converting to glutamine. This process raises intracellular osmotic pressure, leading to cerebral oedema and contributing to the neurological symptoms of hepatic encephalopathy, which can range from mild cognitive changes to coma.

Synthetic failure is another hallmark of liver decompensation. The reduced production of albumin decreases plasma oncotic pressure, causing fluid to shift into the interstitial space and the peritoneal cavity, leading to oedema and ascites. Simultaneously, diminished synthesis of clotting factors, including fibrinogen and vitamin K-dependent proteins, results in coagulopathy and an increased risk of spontaneous or uncontrolled bleeding. In acute cases, impaired gluconeogenesis and depletion of glycogen stores can lead to life-threatening hypoglycaemia, underscoring the liver's vital role in glucose homeostasis.

The accumulation of bilirubin further highlights the liver's central role in metabolism. Impaired conjugation and excretion lead to increased levels of both unconjugated and conjugated bilirubin, resulting in jaundice and dark urine. Cholestasis may also cause pruritus and fat malabsorption, worsening malnutrition in affected patients. At the same time, distortion of the hepatic architecture and increased resistance to portal venous flow cause portal hypertension. This condition leads to complications such as gastro-oesophageal varices, splenomegaly, hypersplenism, and worsening ascites, all of which contribute to morbidity and mortality.

Liver failure also weakens immune defences. Kupffer cells, the liver's resident macrophages, typically clear bacteria and endotoxins from the portal circulation. Their dysfunction, along with reduced complement production, raises susceptibility to infection. Bacterial translocation from the gut is a common occurrence, and patients are at a high risk of developing spontaneous bacterial peritonitis or sepsis.

Ultimately, these processes lead to multi-organ dysfunction. Circulatory changes, characterised by systemic vasodilatation and decreased adequate arterial volume, contribute to renal hypoperfusion and the development of hepatorenal syndrome. Cerebral oedema, worsening encephalopathy, and systemic inflammatory responses can progress to refractory shock and multi-organ failure. Therefore, liver failure not only involves the collapse of a single organ but also triggers a cascade of systemic disturbances that, if unmanaged, are often fatal.

Liver failure occurs when widespread hepatocyte injury hampers the liver's ability to perform its metabolic, synthetic, and detoxifying functions. A key consequence is the build-up of ammonia, which crosses the blood–brain barrier, causes cerebral oedema, and results in hepatic encephalopathy. Synthetic failure leads to decreased production of albumin and clotting factors, resulting in ascites, oedema, and coagulopathy, and, in acute cases, hypoglycaemia due to impaired gluconeogenesis. Disrupted bilirubin metabolism causes jaundice, while distortion of the hepatic vasculature leads to portal hypertension with complications such as varices, splenomegaly, and worsening ascites. Immune dysfunction, driven by diminished Kupffer cell activity and impaired complement synthesis, raises the risk of bacterial translocation and sepsis.

In acute liver failure, these processes happen suddenly, with rapid onset of hypoglycaemia, severe coagulopathy, and cerebral oedema. In chronic liver failure, the underlying issue is progressive fibrosis and architectural distortion, with portal hypertension and malnutrition playing more significant roles. Ultimately, both pathways lead to multi-organ dysfunction, including hepatorenal syndrome, refractory encephalopathy, and circulatory collapse.

Causes

- Acute: paracetamol overdose, viral hepatitis (A, B, and E), autoimmune hepatitis, ischaemic hepatitis, and drug-induced injury.
- Chronic: alcohol-related disease, hepatitis B/C, NAFLD, autoimmune cholangiopathies, haemochromatosis, and Wilson's disease.

Clinical Features

- Early signs: jaundice, fatigue, nausea, and confusion.
- Advanced: encephalopathy, ascites, variceal bleeding, coagulopathy, hepatorenal syndrome, sepsis, hypoglycaemia, and shock.

Investigations

- Liver function tests (LFTs):
  - ALT/AST – hepatocellular injury (ALT is more specific; AST:ALT >2 suggests alcohol).
  - ALP and GGT – indicates cholestasis; GGT confirms hepatic origin and reflects alcohol use.
  - Bilirubin – failure of conjugation/excretion or haemolysis.
  - Albumin – a marker of long-term synthetic function.
  - PT/INR – prolonged in impaired synthetic capacity, a key indicator of severity.
- Other: U&E (renal function), ABG (acidosis), ammonia (encephalopathy), glucose, imaging (USS), and paracentesis if ascites.

Management

- Acute failure: critical care admission, treat cause (e.g. NAC for paracetamol), support (fluids, glucose, infection control), manage complications (encephalopathy, bleeding, renal failure), and early transplant referral (King's criteria).
- Chronic/ACLF: address cause (antivirals, alcohol cessation, immunosuppression), manage ascites with diuretics or paracentesis, use lactulose plus rifaximin for encephalopathy, conduct variceal surveillance and treatment, perform Hepatocellular Carcinoma (HCC) surveillance, and consider transplant for end-stage disease.

Bibliography

British Society of Gastroenterology. Guidelines on the Management of Abnormal Liver Blood Tests. London: BSG; 2018 https://www.bsg.org.uk.

European Association for the Study of the Liver. EASL clinical practice guidelines on the management of decompensated cirrhosis. J Hepatol. 2017;69(2):406–460.

National Institute for Health and Care Excellence. Cirrhosis in Over 16s: Assessment and Management (NG50). London: NICE; 2016, updated 2023. https://www.nice.org.uk

National Institute for Health and Care Excellence. Alcohol-related Liver Disease: Diagnosis and Management (NG49). London: NICE; 2019 https://www.nice.org.uk.

NHS. *Acute liver failure*. 2024. https://www.nhs.uk

Sanyal AJ. Pathogenesis of non-alcoholic fatty liver disease and progression to cirrhosis. Lancet Gastroenterol Hepatol. 2019;4(5):368–379.

Sherlock's Diseases of the Liver and Biliary System. 14th ed. Oxford: Wiley-Blackwell; 2023.

Williams R, Wendon J, Heaton N. Acute liver failure. The Lancet. 2016;388(10044):203–214.

48

Microbiology

Microbiology is the study of microorganisms, including bacteria, viruses, fungi, and parasites, as well as their impact on human health and disease. It forms the foundation of much of modern medicine, from diagnosing and treating infections to creating vaccines and antibiotics. Despite significant advances in prevention and therapy, infections continue to be a major cause of illness and death worldwide.

For clinicians, a practical understanding of microbiology is vital for guiding safe prescribing practices, infection control, and patient care. This chapter offers an overview of key groups of microorganisms, emphasising their structure, clinical significance, and the principles of diagnosis and treatment.

Bacteria

Classification and Structure

Bacteria are prokaryotic organisms characterised by the lack of a nucleus and membrane-bound organelles. They are classified in various ways, most commonly by

- Gram stain reaction
  - Gram-positive bacteria possess thick peptidoglycan cell walls that retain crystal violet (e.g. *Staphylococcus, Streptococcus*).
  - Gram-negative bacteria have thinner cell walls but an extra outer membrane containing lipopolysaccharide (e.g. *Escherichia coli, Pseudomonas aeruginosa*).
- Shape: cocci (spherical), bacilli (rod-shaped), and spirilla/spirochaetes (spiral-shaped).
- Oxygen requirements: aerobic, anaerobic, facultative anaerobes, and microaerophiles.
- Other features: motility (flagella), ability to form spores, and toxin production.

Pathogenic Mechanisms

Bacteria cause disease through a combination of

- Colonisation and invasion of host tissues.
- Production of toxins: exotoxins (protein-based, e.g. tetanus toxin) and endotoxins (lipopolysaccharide from Gram-negative cell walls).
- Evasion of host immunity: capsules, antigenic variation, and biofilm formation.

Clinically Relevant Examples

- Gram-positive cocci
  - *Staphylococcus aureus* causes skin infections, abscesses, pneumonia, and bacteraemia. MRSA is a significant healthcare-associated pathogen.
  - *Streptococcus pneumoniae* – the leading cause of community-acquired pneumonia, meningitis, and otitis media.
  - *Enterococcus species* – normally part of gut flora but can cause urinary tract infections and endocarditis.
- Gram-negative bacilli
  - *E. coli* – a common cause of urinary tract infections, bacteraemia, and gastroenteritis.
  - *Klebsiella pneumoniae* – opportunistic pathogen linked to pneumonia and sepsis, often resistant to multiple drugs.
  - *P. aeruginosa* – causes infections in immunocompromised patients, especially in burns, ventilated patients, and individuals with cystic fibrosis.
- Other significant bacteria
  - *Mycobacterium tuberculosis* causes tuberculosis, a leading cause of infectious death worldwide.
  - *Neisseria meningitidis* – causes meningitis and meningococcaemia, with rapid onset and high mortality.
  - *Clostridium difficile* – causes antibiotic-associated colitis, leading to significant morbidity in hospitalised patients.

Clinical Significance

Bacterial infections continue to be a major cause of hospitalisation and death, especially in low- and middle-income countries. Antibiotics transformed treatment in the twentieth century, but the emergence of antimicrobial resistance (AMR) presents a global health crisis. Understanding bacterial structure and pathogenic mechanisms is essential for guiding effective therapy, infection control, and the development of new treatments.

Viruses

Structure and Classification

Viruses are obligate intracellular parasites, meaning they can only replicate within living host cells. They consist of genetic material (DNA or RNA) enclosed in a protein coat (capsid) and sometimes have an outer lipid envelope. Classification depends on the genome type (DNA vs RNA, single versus double-stranded), the presence or absence of an envelope, and the mode of replication.

Pathogenesis

Viral infection starts when the virus binds to host cell receptors, enters the cell, and hijacks the host's machinery to replicate. Cell damage occurs from direct lysis, immune-mediated harm, or oncogenic transformation. Some viruses enter latency, reactivating under stress or immunosuppression (e.g. herpesviruses).

Clinically Relevant Viruses

- Respiratory viruses: influenza, respiratory syncytial virus (RSV), and SARS-CoV-2.
- Herpesviruses: herpes simplex virus (HSV) causes oral and genital lesions, as well as encephalitis; varicella-zoster virus (VZV) causes chickenpox and shingles.
- Bloodborne viruses: hepatitis B and C viruses cause chronic liver disease and hepatocellular carcinoma; HIV leads to progressive immunodeficiency.
- Childhood viruses: measles, mumps, and rubella – now mostly kept under control by vaccination in developed nations but still widespread in many parts of the world.
- Emerging viruses: Ebola, Zika, and coronaviruses underscore the continued threat of new pathogens and pandemics.

Diagnosis and Treatment

A combination of clinical features, antigen detection, PCR, and serology diagnoses viral infections. Treatment options are limited compared with bacterial infections. Antivirals are available for HIV (antiretrovirals), herpesviruses (acyclovir, ganciclovir), influenza (oseltamivir), and hepatitis viruses. Vaccination remains the most effective tool for prevention.

Fungi

Fungi are eukaryotic organisms that can exist as single-celled yeasts or multicellular moulds. They reproduce through spores and flourish in warm, damp environments. While most fungi are harmless commensals, some cause opportunistic infections, especially in individuals with weakened immune systems.

Classification

- Yeasts: single-celled organisms that reproduce by budding. *Candida* species are the most prevalent, causing oral thrush, vaginal candidiasis, and invasive candidiasis in critically ill patients.
- Moulds: multicellular and filamentous. *Aspergillus* species cause invasive pulmonary aspergillosis, particularly in patients with neutropenia.
- Dimorphic fungi: present as moulds in the environment but as yeasts in human tissue (e.g. *Histoplasma capsulatum*). These are more commonly found in endemic regions outside the United Kingdom.

Pathogenesis

Fungal infections (mycoses) are often opportunistic. Disruption of normal flora (for example, after using broad-spectrum antibiotics) or immune suppression (such as chemotherapy, transplantation, or HIV) increases susceptibility. Invasive disease occurs when fungi penetrate epithelial barriers and spread haematomatically.

Diagnosis and Treatment

Diagnosis may require culture, histopathology, antigen testing (e.g. galactomannan for aspergillosis), or molecular methods. Treatment includes antifungals such as azoles (fluconazole, voriconazole), echinocandins (caspofungin), and amphotericin B. Prophylactic antifungals are often administered to high-risk immunocompromised patients.

Clinical Significance

- *Candida* species are the primary cause of fungal bloodstream infections in hospitals.
- Aspergillus is a major cause of morbidity in recipients of bone marrow and solid organ transplants.
- Endemic mycoses such as histoplasmosis and coccidioidomycosis are uncommon in the United Kingdom but should be considered in travellers.

Parasites

Parasites include protozoa, helminths, and ectoparasites, many of which cause significant diseases worldwide.

- Protozoa: *Plasmodium* species cause malaria, which remains one of the world's leading infectious killers. *Toxoplasma gondii* can cause severe disease in pregnancy or immunosuppressed patients.
- Helminths: worms such as *Schistosoma* and *Ascaris* contribute to chronic morbidity in endemic areas.
- Ectoparasites: lice, fleas, and ticks can directly cause disease and transmit bacterial or viral infections.

In the United Kingdom, parasitic infections are relatively uncommon but should be considered in travellers, migrants, and immunocompromised patients.

Bibliography

Davidson's Principles and Practice of Medicine. 24th ed. Edinburgh: Elsevier; 2022.
European Centre for Disease Prevention and Control. Surveillance of Infectious Diseases in Europe. Stockholm: ECDC; 2024 https://www.ecdc.europa.eu.
Jawetz, Melnick & Adelberg's Medical Microbiology. 29th ed. New York: McGraw-Hill; 2022.
Medical Microbiology. 10th ed. Philadelphia: Elsevier; 2023.

Mims' Medical Microbiology and Immunology. 7th ed. Edinburgh: Elsevier; 2024.

National Institute for Health and Care Excellence. Antimicrobial Stewardship: Systems and Processes for Effective Antimicrobial Medicine use (NG15). London: NICE; 2023 https://www.nice.org.uk.

Oxford Handbook of Infectious Diseases and Microbiology. 3rd ed. Oxford: Oxford University Press; 2023.

Sherris Medical Microbiology. 8th ed. New York: McGraw-Hill; 2023.

UK Health Security Agency. Infectious Diseases and Microbiology Guidance. London: UKHSA; 2024 https://www.gov.uk/ukhsa.

World Health Organization. Antimicrobial Resistance: Global Report on Surveillance. Geneva: WHO; 2023 https://www.who.int.

49

Necrotising Fasciitis

Necrotising fasciitis (NF) is a rapidly progressing, life-threatening soft tissue infection characterised by extensive fascial necrosis with relatively sparing of skin and muscle in early stages. It spreads along fascial planes, leading to vascular thrombosis, tissue ischaemia, and systemic illness caused by toxins. Without prompt recognition and treatment, mortality remains high.

Pathophysiology

Infection usually follows trauma, surgery, or IV drug use, though it can arise spontaneously. The poorly vascularised fascia provides little immune defence, allowing bacteria (often Group A Streptococcus or polymicrobial flora) to proliferate unchecked. Exotoxins and enzymes accelerate tissue destruction and trigger systemic inflammatory response, leading to septic shock and multi-organ failure.

Classification

- Type I (polymicrobial): aerobes + anaerobes, common in diabetes or immunocompromised patients.
- Type II (monomicrobial): usually caused by Group A Streptococcus ± *Staphylococcus aureus*, affecting healthy individuals.
- Type III: *Vibrio vulnificus* (exposure to seawater).
- Type IV: rare fungal infections in immunosuppressed individuals.

Clinical Features

- Early: severe pain disproportionate to findings, erythema, and swelling.
- Progression: dusky discolouration, bullae, subcutaneous crepitus, and systemic toxicity (fever, tachycardia, hypotension).
- Late: septic shock, multiple organ dysfunction, and disseminated intravascular coagulation (DIC).

Diagnosis

NF is primarily a clinical diagnosis – do not delay surgery for tests.

- Bloods: ↑ CRP, WCC, CK, and lactate; hyponatraemia common.
- Imaging: CT/MRI can assist diagnosis but must not delay theatre.
- Operative findings: grey 'dishwater' fluid, friable fascia, and absence of bleeding.

Management

- Surgical emergency: immediate, aggressive debridement with possible repeat operations.
- Antibiotics: broad spectrum (e.g. meropenem + clindamycin + vancomycin), adjusted once sensitivities are known.
- Supportive care: HDU/ICU admission, fluids, vasopressors, and renal support if necessary.

Prognosis

Mortality rates range from 20% to 40% and are higher with delayed diagnosis or comorbidities. Survival hinges on early recognition, prompt surgery, and comprehensive critical care.

Bibliography

Ardehali B, Khan U. Necrotizing fasciitis. In: Aziz O, Purkayastha S, Paraskevas P, eds. Hospital Surgery: Foundations in Surgical Practice. Cambridge: Cambridge University Press; 2009, pp. 308–311.

British Association of Plastic, Reconstructive and Aesthetic Surgeons. Guidance on the Management of Necrotising Soft Tissue Infections. London: BAPRAS; 2022 https://www.bapras.org.uk.

Mims' Medical Microbiology and Immunology. 7th ed. Edinburgh: Elsevier; 2024.

National Institute for Health and Care Excellence. Sepsis: Recognition, Diagnosis and Early Management (NG51). London: NICE; 2020 https://www.nice.org.uk.

Sawyer RG, McLean EAB. Necrotizing fasciitis and other soft tissue infections. Lancet Infect Dis. 2020;20(5):600–612.

Stevens DL, Bryant AE, Bisno AE. Necrotizing soft-tissue infections. N Engl J Med. 2017;377(23):2253–2265.

UK Health Security Agency. Group A Streptococcal Infections: Epidemiology, Management and Prevention. London: UKHSA; 2024 https://www.gov.uk/ukhsa.

50

Nutrition Overview

Nutrition is a vital part of patient care in hospital environments. Adequate nutritional intake assists wound healing, immune function, tissue repair, and overall recovery. Malnutrition – whether caused by chronic illness, acute disease, or hospital-related underfeeding – is linked to increased morbidity, longer hospital stays, and higher mortality.

Hospitalised patients often have increased metabolic demands (e.g. in sepsis, trauma, burns) and decreased intake (e.g. due to nausea, dysphagia, reduced consciousness, or mechanical ventilation). Early nutritional screening (e.g. using the MUST score) helps identify those at risk and enables timely intervention.

Basic Nutritional Requirements

Although needs differ among individuals, general estimates for adult hospitalised patients are:

- Calories: 25–30 kcal/kg/day.
- Protein: 1.2–2 g/kg/day (higher in catabolic states such as trauma or sepsis).
- Fluid: 30–35 mL/kg/day (adjusted for losses, comorbidities).
- Micronutrients: adequate vitamins and trace elements are vital, especially during prolonged illness or refeeding (ESPEN, 2019).

Routes of Nutrition

Oral Nutrition

First-line treatment if safe and tolerated. This includes regular diets with fortified meals, oral nutritional supplements (ONS), or texture-modified diets for swallowing difficulties.

Enteral Feeding

Enteral feeding is preferred when oral intake is insufficient but the gut remains functional.

- Nasogastric (NG) tube: for short-term use; requires confirmation of placement.
- Nasojejunal (NJ) tube: used for intolerance to gastric feeding.
- PEG feeding: long-term access (>4 weeks), inserted endoscopically or surgically.

Parenteral Nutrition (TPN)

Parenteral nutrition (TPN) is reserved for when the gastrointestinal (GI) tract is non-functional or unsafe. It is administered via a central line and requires careful biochemical and clinical monitoring due to risks such as line sepsis, liver dysfunction, and refeeding syndrome.

Monitoring and Complications

Daily monitoring covers nutritional intake, weight, and fluid balance, along with blood tests (U&Es, glucose, liver function, electrolytes). Special attention is needed for refeeding syndrome (characterised by hypophosphataemia, hypokalaemia, and hypomagnesaemia), which can be life-threatening if not anticipated and managed properly. Feeding plans should be regularly adjusted based on clinical progress and tolerance.

Bibliography

BAPEN. The ‘MUST’ Explanatory Booklet. British Association for Parenteral and Enteral Nutrition; 2011.

Correia MITD, Waitzberg DL. The impact of malnutrition on morbidity, mortality, length of hospital stay and costs evaluated through a multivariate model analysis. Clin Nutr. 2003;22(3):235–239.

ESPEN. ESPEN guideline on clinical nutrition in the intensive care unit. Clin Nutr. 2019;38(1):48–79.

NICE. Nutrition Support for Adults: Oral Nutrition Support, Enteral Tube Feeding and Parenteral Nutrition (CG32). National Institute for Health and Care Excellence; 2006.

NICE. Nutrition Support in Adults: Quality Standard (QS24). National Institute for Health and Care Excellence; 2017.

51

Ophthalmology Overview

Ophthalmic conditions can occur as stand-alone problems or as signs of systemic disease. Recognising red flag symptoms is essential, as some eye conditions can quickly result in irreversible vision loss or indicate life-threatening issues.

Red Flag Symptoms

Urgent ophthalmology review needed for

- Sudden loss of vision (painful or painless).
- Painful red eye with photophobia or reduced vision.
- Flashes, floaters, or 'curtain-like' visual loss.
- New diplopia (especially with neurological signs).
- Chemical injuries.
- Penetrating trauma or high-risk foreign bodies.

Common Presentations

- Conjunctivitis
  - Bacterial: unilateral and sticky discharge → topical antibiotics.
  - Viral: bilateral, watery, and highly contagious → supportive care.
  - Allergic: itchy and often bilateral → antihistamines/mast cell stabilisers.
- Corneal abrasion
  - Trauma/contact lens-related; painful and photophobia.
  - Fluorescein staining confirms.
  - Treat with topical antibiotics and analgesia; never patch.
- Acute angle-closure glaucoma
  - Painful red eye, blurred vision, haloes, nausea, and fixed mid-dilated pupil.
  - Ophthalmic emergency → acetazolamide, pilocarpine, and urgent referral.

- Orbital cellulitis
  - Pain, swelling, ophthalmoplegia, and systemic illness.
  - Requires IV antibiotics + urgent ophthalmology/ENT input.
- Retinal detachment
  - Flashes, floaters, 'curtain' over vision, and painless.
  - Immediate surgical referral.
- Temporal arteritis (giant cell arteritis)
  - Age > 50, headache, scalp tenderness, jaw claudication, and visual disturbance.
  - Start high-dose steroids immediately, urgent referral.

Basic Examination

- Always document visual acuity (Snellen or bedside).
- Pupils – equality, reactivity, and relative afferent pupillary defect (RAPD).
- Visual fields – confrontation testing.
- Ocular movements – diplopia/restriction.
- External eye – redness, swelling, and discharge.
- Fundoscopy – optic disc, vessels if possible.

Bibliography

BMJ Best Practice. Red Eye in Adults. BMJ Publishing Group; 2023.

National Institute for Health and Care Excellence (NICE). Glaucoma: Diagnosis and Management. NG81; 2022.

Royal College of Ophthalmologists. Clinical Guidelines. RCOphth; 2020.

Salmon JF, Kanski JJ. Clinical Ophthalmology: A Systematic Approach. 9th ed. Elsevier; 2020.

52

Organ Donation

Advanced practitioners play a vital role in supporting organ donation. Donations can occur in two ways: donation after brain stem death (DBD), which follows a diagnosis of death via neurological criteria, formally known as brain stem death testing, or donation after circulatory death (DCD). A Specialist Nurse in Organ Donation (SN-OD) must be notified early when the medical team has decided to withdraw life-sustaining treatment or has recognised that testing for neurological death should be performed.

Early notification enables effective teamwork. The SN-OD's role includes verifying the suitability for donation, exploring patients' prior donation decisions, supporting donor management and optimisation, coordinating with involved teams, and organising the donation process. A consultant is responsible for leading the decision and discussion about withdrawing treatment, although the SN-OD usually leads the conversation about donation.

In DCD, the patient is transferred to the theatre for organ retrieval, typically after life-sustaining treatment has been withdrawn in the anaesthetic room. Once asystole is confirmed and death is established, the patient is moved to the operating theatre for organ retrieval. Death must occur within a three to four-hour window and in a manner that maintains organ quality. If death does not occur within this timeframe, the patient will be returned to the critical care unit for ongoing palliative care; tissue donation can still proceed.

The diagnosis of death via neurological criteria must be performed by two senior doctors, including at least one consultant. Two sets of tests are required, with the first set providing the date and time of death. Patients must be stabilised and optimised, with preconditions such as a primary diagnosis of irreversible brain damage, a Glasgow Coma Score (GCS) of 3, being mechanically ventilated, and the exclusion of reversible causes of coma and apnoea, to ensure no residual effects of sedation or neuromuscular blockade, to be considered suitable for testing. Brain stem tests and cranial nerve assessments are also crucial.

Brain Stem Tests and Cranial Nerves

Test	Cranial Nerve(s)	Method	Expected Response
Pupillary light reflex	II, III	Shine light into each eye	Pupils constrict
Corneal reflex	V, VII	Touch cornea with cotton wool	Blink response
Oculocephalic reflex (Doll's eye manoeuvre)	III, IV, VI, VIII	Rotate head rapidly side to side	Eyes move in opposite direction (if brain stem intact)
Oculovestibular reflex (caloric test)	III, VI, VIII	Ice-cold water into external auditory canal	Eye deviation towards irrigated ear
Gag reflex	IX, X	Stimulate posterior pharynx	Pharyngeal movement/ gag
Cough reflex	X	Pass a suction catheter into the trachea/bronchi	Coughing or movement
Apnoea test	Brain stem integrative function	Disconnect the ventilator after pre-oxygenation, monitor for spontaneous breaths with rising $PaCO_2$	No respiratory effort

Management

National protocols direct the management of potential organ donors to ensure organs are preserved in the best condition for transplantation. In the United Kingdom, this involves a structured, multidisciplinary approach once consent or authorisation for donation has been granted. Donor optimisation seeks to maintain adequate organ perfusion, oxygen delivery, and metabolic stability, as physiological deterioration after brain stem death or circulatory death can compromise organ quality.

Key parameters are carefully monitored and adjusted. Haemodynamic stability is maintained with a mean arterial pressure of 65–90 mmHg using intravenous fluids and vasopressors as needed. Oxygenation is optimised with a target PaO_2 above 10 kPa and oxygen saturations above 95%, while ventilation strategies aim to prevent volutrauma and keep $PaCO_2$ within the normal range. Temperature is maintained above 35 °C to avoid coagulopathy and metabolic disturbances, and blood glucose is regulated between 4 and 10 mmol/L. Electrolyte levels, especially potassium and sodium, are corrected, and urine output is observed at 0.5–2 mL/kg/hr to indicate adequate renal perfusion. Hormonal resuscitation, including vasopressin, corticosteroids, and insulin, may be given according to local protocols to support cardiovascular stability and reduce inflammatory injury.

These interventions are coordinated by the critical care team in collaboration with NHS Blood and Transplant donor coordinators. Regular reassessment and documentation ensure that organs are preserved in optimal condition until retrieval. The process requires not only adherence to physiological targets but also sensitive communication with families, respect for the donor, and close liaison with retrieval teams to maximise successful transplantation outcomes.

Bibliography

Academy of Medical Royal Colleges. A Code of Practice for the Diagnosis and Confirmation of Death. London: AoMRC; 2008.

NHS Blood and Transplant. Organ Donation and Transplantation Clinical Guidelines. NHSBT; 2020.

Wijdicks EFM. Brain death. N Engl J Med. 2001;344:1215–1221.

53

Common Toxicological Emergencies

Paracetamol (Acetaminophen)

Paracetamol is metabolised in the liver mainly through glucuronidation and sulphation. A small proportion is transformed into the toxic metabolite N-acetyl-p-benzoquinone imine (NAPQI). Under normal conditions, NAPQI is detoxified by glutathione, but during an overdose, glutathione reserves become depleted, allowing NAPQI to accumulate and cause hepatocellular necrosis.

Management involves administering activated charcoal if the patient presents within one hour of ingestion, and giving N-acetylcysteine (NAC) based on paracetamol levels and timing. Liver function tests, International Normalised Ratio (INR), and renal function should be monitored, and referral to a specialist liver unit may be required in severe cases.

Aspirin (Salicylates)

Salicylates stimulate the respiratory centre, initially causing a primary respiratory alkalosis. This is followed by a high anion gap metabolic acidosis due to impaired oxidative phosphorylation. Severe toxicity can result in cerebral oedema, seizures, and death.

Management involves early administration of activated charcoal, correction of hypokalaemia, and urinary alkalinisation with intravenous sodium bicarbonate to promote excretion. Haemodialysis is recommended in severe poisoning, for example, when salicylate levels exceed 500 mg/L or if there is significant acidosis or renal impairment.

Opioids

Opioids bind to μ-opioid receptors, depressing the central nervous system and inhibiting brainstem respiratory centres. This results in hypoventilation, hypoxia, and an increased risk of death without intervention.

Management requires airway support and assisted ventilation if necessary. Naloxone can be administered intravenously, intramuscularly, or intranasally, to restore adequate respiratory effort rather than full consciousness. Due to naloxone's short half-life, repeated doses or continuous infusion may be required.

Benzodiazepines

Benzodiazepines enhance gamma-aminobutyric acid (GABA)"s effect at the GABA-A receptor by increasing chloride influx, leading to central nervous system depression. Overdose is rarely life-threatening unless combined with other depressants such as alcohol or opioids.

Management is mainly supportive, with airway protection as necessary. Flumazenil may be considered in cases of isolated benzodiazepine overdose with no risk of co-ingestants or dependence, but its use carries a risk of triggering seizures.

Tricyclic Antidepressants (TCAs)

Tricyclic antidepressants (TCAs) cause toxic effects by blocking sodium channels, anticholinergic receptors, and GABA receptors. Overdose may lead to cardiac conduction delays with prolonged QRS intervals, seizures, hypotension, and life-threatening arrhythmias.

Management includes administering intravenous sodium bicarbonate to narrow QRS complexes and correct acidosis. Seizures are treated with benzodiazepines. Continuous ECG and electrolyte monitoring are essential.

Beta-blockers

In overdose, beta-blockers decrease heart rate and myocardial contractility by antagonising β1 receptors, leading to bradycardia, hypotension, heart block, and, in severe cases, cardiogenic shock.

Management includes intravenous atropine, glucagon, and calcium gluconate. Refractory cases may require high-dose insulin euglycaemic therapy (HIET), vasopressors, or temporary pacing.

Calcium Channel Blockers (CCBs)

Calcium channel blockers (CCBs) inhibit L-type calcium channels, decreasing cardiac contractility and causing vasodilation. Overdose usually presents with bradycardia, hypotension, and sometimes hyperglycaemia due to impaired insulin secretion.

Treatment includes intravenous calcium gluconate, high-dose insulin therapy, and supportive fluids. Vasopressors such as noradrenaline may be necessary, with close monitoring of glucose and potassium levels.

Iron

Iron poisoning progresses through stages: initial gastrointestinal symptoms, a temporary quiescent phase, and later systemic toxicity with metabolic acidosis, hepatic failure, and coagulopathy. Free iron exerts direct cellular toxicity and disrupts oxidative phosphorylation.

Management involves checking serum iron levels. Deferoxamine chelation is indicated if serum concentrations exceed 90 μmol/L or if systemic features are present. Supportive measures include intravenous fluids and correction of acidosis.

Lithium

Lithium toxicity impacts both the central nervous system and the kidneys. It interferes with neurotransmission, causing tremor, confusion, ataxia, and seizures. Renal toxicity may present as nephrogenic diabetes insipidus.

Management involves discontinuing lithium and rehydrating with intravenous fluids to improve renal clearance. Severe cases or those with renal impairment require haemodialysis, especially if serum lithium exceeds 4.0 mmol/L or 2.5 mmol/L in the presence of symptoms.

Alcohols (Ethanol, Methanol, and Ethylene Glycol)

Methanol and ethylene glycol are metabolised by alcohol dehydrogenase into toxic metabolites, formic acid and oxalic acid, which cause metabolic acidosis, retinal toxicity, and renal failure.

Treatment involves administering fomepizole, or ethanol if unavailable, to competitively inhibit alcohol dehydrogenase. Haemodialysis may be necessary in severe poisoning to remove the parent alcohol and its metabolites. Intravenous bicarbonate is employed to correct acidosis.

Organophosphates

Organophosphate poisoning occurs due to inhibition of acetylcholinesterase, resulting in an accumulation of acetylcholine at synapses. This causes a cholinergic crisis, characterised by salivation, lacrimation, urination, diarrhoea, gastrointestinal upset, vomiting, bradycardia, bronchorrhoea, and muscle fasciculations.

Management includes decontaminating the patient and safeguarding healthcare workers from exposure. Atropine is administered to counteract muscarinic effects, and pralidoxime is used to regenerate acetylcholinesterase.

Bibliography

Bateman DN, Dear JW. Paracetamol (acetaminophen) poisoning. N Engl J Med. 2016;375:1111–1121.

BMJ Best Practice. Poisoning – Overview and Management. BMJ Publishing Group; 2025.

LITFL (Life in the Fast Lane). Toxicology clinical resources. n.d.

National Institute for Health and Care Excellence (NICE). Paracetamol overdose: diagnosis, assessment and management. 2019.

National Poisons Information Service (NPIS). TOXBASE clinical toxicology database. https://www.toxbase.org. n.d.

Resuscitation Council UK. Medical emergencies and toxicological emergencies guidelines. 2025

Vale JA, Bradberry SM. Poisoning and overdose. In: Oxford Handbook of Acute Medicine. 3rd ed. Oxford University Press; 2020.

54

Overview of Medical Imaging

Medical imaging underpins modern diagnosis and management. Each modality has unique strengths and limitations; selecting the appropriate test enhances safety and diagnostic accuracy.

Modality	Principle	Main Uses	Advantages	Limitations
X-ray	Ionising radiation and 2D image	Bone fractures, chest disease, and foreign bodies	Fast, cheap, and widely available	Limited soft tissue detail and radiation
CT	Rotating X-ray beams → cross-sectional images	Trauma, stroke, cancer staging, and chest/abdo pathology	High detail, fast, and 3D reconstruction	High radiation and less soft tissue contrast
MRI	Magnetic fields + radiofrequency	Brain/spine, joints, cardiac, and soft tissue tumours	Excellent soft tissue contrast and no ionising radiation	Expensive, time-consuming, and contraindications (implants, claustrophobia)
Ultrasound	High-frequency sound waves	Abdomen, obstetrics, vascular, and procedural guidance	Portable, safe, real time, and no radiation	Operator dependent and limited by bone/gas
Nuclear medicine (PET/SPECT)	Radiotracers emit gamma rays	Oncology staging, cardiac perfusion, and dementia imaging	Functional + metabolic imaging and early disease detection	Radiation and poor anatomical detail (often combined with CT)
Fluoroscopy	Continuous X-ray and real-time imaging	GI studies, catheter/line placement, and joint injections	Dynamic studies and procedural guidance	Radiation exposure and limited soft tissue detail

Bibliography

The Royal College of Radiologists. iRefer: Making the Best Use of Clinical Radiology. 9th ed. RCR; 2022.

NICE. Suspected Cancer: Recognition and Referral (NG12). National Institute for Health and Care Excellence; 2023.

NICE. Stroke and Transient Ischaemic Attack in Over 16s: Diagnosis and Initial Management (NG128). NICE; 2019.

NHS England. Clinical Imaging: Guidance for Clinicians. NHS England; 2022.

55

Palliative Care

Palliative care is a holistic, multidisciplinary approach aimed at improving the quality of life for individuals living with a life-limiting illness and their families. The WHO defines it as care that seeks to prevent and relieve suffering through early identification, assessment, and management of pain and other issues – physical, psychosocial, and spiritual. Palliative care is not confined to the final days of life; it can and should be introduced early during progressive conditions such as cancer, advanced heart failure, chronic obstructive pulmonary disease (COPD), dementia, and motor neurone disease, alongside disease-modifying or life-prolonging treatments.

Core Principles

- Symptom management: relief of pain, dyspnoea, nausea, agitation, constipation, fatigue, and other distressing symptoms.
- Holistic care: recognising that suffering is multidimensional – physical, psychological, social, and spiritual.
- Patient-centred decision-making: encouraging open discussions about preferences, values, and care goals, including advance care planning and treatment escalation decisions (e.g. do not attempt cardiopulmonary resuscitation [DNACPR] orders, Recommended Summary Plan for Emergency Care and Treatment [ReSPECT] forms).
- Family support: emotional, practical, and bereavement assistance for relatives and carers.
- Dignity in dying: aiding a peaceful, respectful death in the setting preferred by the patient whenever possible.

The Holistic Model of Care

- Physical: disease burden, treatment side effects, and increasing frailty.
- Psychological: fear, anxiety, depression, or existential distress.
- Social: influence on roles, relationships, employment, and finances.
- Spiritual/existential: seeking meaning, faith, hope, or peace.

This model recognises that high-quality palliative care must address all these dimensions simultaneously, often requiring input from a multidisciplinary team.

Providers of Palliative Care

Generalist palliative care: provided by all healthcare professionals in primary and secondary care, concentrating on basic symptom relief and effective communication.

Specialist palliative care: delivered by dedicated teams including consultants, clinical nurse specialists, allied health professionals, social workers, and chaplains when symptoms are complex, refractory, or require advanced interventions.

Common Symptoms and Their Management

- Pain: follow the WHO analgesic ladder; titrate opioids carefully while considering adjuvant therapies (e.g. neuropathic pain agents).
- Nausea and vomiting: determine the underlying cause; haloperidol (chemical causes), cyclizine (raised intra-cranial pressure [ICP], or ondansetron (gut obstruction/chemotherapy).
- Dyspnoea: low-dose opioids can ease breathlessness. Non-pharmacological measures (open window, handheld fan, positioning) are also effective. Oxygen is reserved for hypoxaemic patients.
- Delirium and agitation: assess for reversible causes, but use haloperidol or midazolam for symptomatic relief.
- Terminal respiratory secretions ('death rattle'): anticholinergics (e.g. glycopyrronium, hyoscine butylbromide) reduce distressing noise but are not always necessary for comfort.

End-of-Life Care (Last Days of Life)

When death is expected within days, the focus shifts entirely to comfort and dignity.

- Discontinue non-essential medications and burdensome interventions.
- Prescribe anticipatory medications for pain, agitation, breathlessness, nausea, and secretions.
- Review hydration and nutrition to align with comfort and care objectives.
- Communicate honestly and compassionately with families about the dying process.
- Ensure a coordinated, documented plan (e.g. ReSPECT or local treatment escalation planning).

Summary

Palliative care is about more than just dying well; it is about helping people live well despite serious illness. Through timely, person-centred, and holistic support, patients and families can experience an improved quality of life, fewer symptoms, and greater dignity at the end of life.

Bibliography

National Institute for Health and Care Excellence (NICE). End of Life Care for Adults: Service Delivery (NG142). London: NICE; 2019.

National Palliative and End of Life Care Partnership. Ambitions for Palliative and End of Life Care: A National Framework for Local Action 2021–2026. London: NHS England; 2021.

Twycross R, Wilcock A, Howard P. Palliative Care Formulary. 7th ed. London: Pharmaceutical Press; 2023.

World Health Organization. Palliative Care. Geneva: WHO; 2020.

56

Pancreatitis

Pancreatitis is an inflammation of the pancreas, usually divided into two forms: acute and chronic. The pancreas has both endocrine and exocrine functions, and damage can interfere with digestion, glucose control, and overall bodily balance. Acute pancreatitis is a common emergency, ranging from mild, self-limiting disease to severe necrotising pancreatitis with multiple organ failure.

Pathophysiology

Acute pancreatitis occurs due to premature activation of digestive enzymes, especially trypsin, within the pancreatic acinar cells. Instead of being secreted into the duodenum, these enzymes cause autodigestion of pancreatic tissue, leading to oedema, necrosis, and haemorrhage. Fat necrosis is caused by lipase activity, while elastase damages blood vessels, resulting in haemorrhage. The release of cytokines (IL-1, IL-6, TNF-α) enhances the inflammatory cascade, which can sometimes result in systemic inflammatory response syndrome (SIRS) and multi-organ dysfunction.

Chronic pancreatitis occurs when repeated inflammation causes fibrosis, calcification, and permanent damage. This leads to loss of exocrine function (steatorrhoea, malabsorption) and eventually results in endocrine failure (diabetes mellitus).

Causes

- Gallstones – ductal obstruction
- Alcohol – toxic effect on acinar cells
- Hypertriglyceridaemia
- Drugs (e.g. azathioprine, thiazides)
- Endoscopic retrograde cholangiopancreatography (ERCP) and trauma
- Autoimmune or idiopathic
- Viral infections (e.g. mumps)

Clinical Features

- Severe, sudden epigastric pain radiating to the back.
- Nausea, vomiting, and abdominal tenderness.
- Systemic: tachycardia, hypotension, fever, and jaundice.
- Rare signs of haemorrhagic pancreatitis: Cullen's sign (periumbilical bruising) and Grey–Turner's sign (flank bruising).

Investigations

- Serum amylase or lipase – lipase is more specific.
- FBC, U&Es, and CRP – assess inflammation and organ function.
- LFTs – suggest gallstone aetiology.
- Ultrasound – gallstones and biliary dilatation.
- CT abdomen – assess complications/necrosis if severe or unclear.

Management

- Supportive: aggressive IV fluids (first 24 hours crucial), opioid analgesia, oxygen, and electrolyte correction.
- Nil by mouth initially; NG tube if persistent vomiting.
- ERCP in cases of gallstone pancreatitis with cholangitis or biliary obstruction.
- Antibiotics only if evidence of infected necrosis or sepsis

Complications

Early: shock, acute respiratory distress syndrome (ARDS) renal failure, necrosis, and SIRS.
Late: pseudocyst, abscess, and chronic pancreatitis with exocrine and endocrine insufficiency.

Chronic Pancreatitis

Typically alcohol-related. Features include chronic pain, steatorrhoea, and diabetes. Management involves enzyme replacement, dietary modification, and analgesia.

Bibliography

Banks PA, Bollen TL, Dervenis C, et al. Classification of acute pancreatitis—2012: revision of the Atlanta classification and definitions by international consensus. Gut. 2013;62(1):102–111.

NICE. Pancreatitis: Diagnosis and Management [NG104]. National Institute for Health and Care Excellence; 2018.

Petrov MS, Yadav D. Global epidemiology and holistic prevention of pancreatitis. Nat Rev Gastroenterol Hepatol. 2019;16(3):175–184.

Tenner S, Baillie J, DeWitt J, Vege SS. American College of Gastroenterology guideline: management of acute pancreatitis. Am J Gastroenterol. 2013;108(9):1400–1415.

57

Pneumonia

Pneumonia is an acute infection of the lung tissue, leading to inflammation and consolidation of the alveoli. It can be classified as community-acquired pneumonia (CAP), hospital-acquired pneumonia (HAP), or ventilator-associated pneumonia (VAP). It remains a significant cause of morbidity and mortality worldwide, especially in older adults and patients with comorbidities.

Pathophysiology

Under normal conditions, the respiratory tract is protected by mucociliary clearance, secretory IgA, alveolar macrophages, and an intact cough reflex. When these defences are breached – through inhalation of pathogens, aspiration of secretions, or haematogenous spread – microorganisms invade the alveoli. This triggers a local immune response, characterised by the recruitment of neutrophils and the release of cytokines. Alveoli fill with inflammatory exudate, impairing oxygen diffusion and causing hypoxaemia.

Traditionally, bacterial pneumonia advances through four histological stages.

1) Congestion – vascular engorgement and proteinaceous exudate in the alveoli.
2) Red hepatisation – alveoli packed with neutrophils, fibrin, and red blood cells.
3) Grey hepatisation – breakdown of red cells and retention of fibrinous exudate.
4) Resolution – enzymatic breakdown of exudate and restoration of normal tissue structure.

In viral or atypical pneumonias, the pattern is more interstitial, featuring lymphocytic infiltration and less consolidation.

Common Causes

- CAP: *Streptococcus pneumoniae* (most common), *Haemophilus influenzae*, *Mycoplasma pneumoniae*, *Legionella pneumophila*, and respiratory viruses (e.g. influenza, SARS-CoV-2).

- HAP: Gram-negative bacilli (*Pseudomonas aeruginosa*, *Klebsiella pneumoniae*) and *Staphylococcus aureus* (including MRSA).
- Aspiration pneumonia: anaerobes from the oropharynx (e.g. *Bacteroides*, *Fusobacterium*) are common in individuals with reduced consciousness or dysphagia.
- Immunocompromised: fungi (*Pneumocystis jirovecii*, Aspergillus), Cytomegalovirus and *Mycobacterium tuberculosis*.

Clinical Features

- Cough, often producing purulent or rusty sputum.
- Fever, rigours, and malaise.
- Dyspnoea, tachypnoea, and hypoxia.
- Pleuritic chest pain.
- Auscultation: crepitations, bronchial breathing, and reduced air entry.
- Elderly patients may present atypically, such as confusion, falls, or anorexia.

Investigations

- Chext X-Ray: lobar consolidation (typical bacterial pneumonia) or patchy infiltrates (atypical/viral).
- Bloods: elevated WCC and CRP; U&Es to evaluate hydration and kidney function.
- Microbiology: blood cultures, sputum culture, and urinary antigens (e.g. *Legionella*, pneumococcus).
- ABG: indicated if hypoxic, tachypnoeic, or with altered consciousness.
- Severity assessment: CURB-65 score (Confusion, Urea > 7, RR ≥ 30, BP < 90 systolic or ≤60 diastolic, age ≥ 65) guides treatment and hospitalisation decisions.

Management

- Supportive care: oxygen for hypoxia, IV fluids for dehydration, analgesia, and antipyretics.
- Antibiotics (local policy may differ)
  - Mild CAP: oral amoxicillin, doxycycline, or clarithromycin.
  - Moderate to severe CAP: IV co-amoxiclav with clarithromycin.
  - HAP/VAP: broad-spectrum antibiotics (e.g. piperacillin–tazobactam, meropenem, or as determined by microbiology).
- Physiotherapy: chest physiotherapy and mobilisation for hospitalised patients.
- Venous thromboembolismprophylaxis: administered if immobile and no contraindications.
- Follow-up CXR: at 6–8 weeks in high-risk patients (e.g. smokers, unresolved symptoms) to exclude underlying malignancy.

Complications

Complications of pneumonia occur when the inflammatory response extends beyond the alveoli or when infection is not adequately controlled. A common complication is a parapneumonic effusion, where fluid accumulates in the pleural space. If bacterial invasion occurs, this can progress to empyema, requiring drainage and prolonged antibiotics. Localised infection may also lead to lung abscess formation, characterised by cavitation, necrosis, and persistent fever. These structural complications not only prolong recovery but may also predispose to chronic lung disease if not managed effectively.

Systemic consequences can be equally severe. Severe pneumonia may lead to sepsis, with widespread inflammatory activation causing hypotension, multi-organ failure, and sometimes death. Inflammation in the lungs can also trigger acute respiratory distress syndrome (ARDS), characterised by diffuse alveolar damage, severe hypoxaemia, and the need for ventilatory support. Long-term effects are increasingly recognised, especially in patients with recurrent or severe infections. These include post-infectious bronchiectasis, where permanent dilatation of the bronchi results in chronic cough and sputum production, or pulmonary fibrosis, which leads to restrictive lung disease and reduced exercise capacity. Overall, these complications emphasise the importance of early detection and prompt treatment of pneumonia to reduce both immediate and long-term morbidity.

Bibliography

British Thoracic Society (BTS). Guidelines for the management of community-acquired pneumonia in adults: update 2009. Thorax. 2009;64(Suppl 3):iii1–iii55.

Mandell LA, Niederman MS. Aspiration pneumonia. N Engl J Med. 2019;380(7):651–663.

Metlay JP, Waterer GW, Long AC, et al. Diagnosis and treatment of adults with community-acquired pneumonia. Am J Respir Crit Care Med. 2019;200(7):e45–e67.

National Institute for Health and Care Excellence (NICE). Pneumonia in Adults: Diagnosis and Management. NG138; 2019.

58

Pneumothorax

A pneumothorax is the presence of air in the pleural space, causing the lung to partially or completely collapse. It can occur spontaneously, due to lung disease, or as a result of trauma or medical intervention. Severity depends on the size and extent of cardiorespiratory disturbance.

Pathophysiology

The pleural space normally maintains negative pressure, keeping the lungs expanded. Air entry, either through alveolar rupture or trauma, disrupts this, allowing the lung to recoil and collapse. Gas exchange is impaired, leading to hypoxia. In tension pneumothorax, a one-way valve effect traps air, increasing intrathoracic pressure, shifting the mediastinum, and blocking venous return – quickly resulting in shock and death if not treated.

Types

- Primary spontaneous: tall, slender young men; rupture of subpleural blebs.
- Secondary spontaneous: underlying lung disease (e.g. COPD, asthma, TB, malignancy).
- Traumatic: blunt or penetrating injury; iatrogenic (central line, ventilation).
- Tension: emergency; increasing pressure compresses the mediastinum, leading to shock.

Clinical Features

- Sudden pleuritic chest pain.
- Dyspnoea (mild to severe).
- Diminished breath sounds, hyperresonance, and decreased chest expansion.
- Signs of tension: tracheal deviation, JVP distension, hypotension, and cyanosis.

Investigations

- Chest X-Ray: visible pleural line, absent lung markings beyond; mediastinal shift due to tension.

- CT: more sensitive, particularly in trauma.
- Ultrasound: absence of pleural sliding ('lung point') in trauma/point of care ultrasound

Management

- Small, stable primary: observation + O_2.
- Needle aspiration: first line in larger or symptomatic primary pneumothoraces.
- Chest drain: if aspiration fails, in secondary pneumothorax, or if unstable.
- Tension pneumothorax: immediate needle decompression (2nd ICS, midclavicular) → chest drain (5th ICS, midaxillary).
- Surgery (video-assisted thoracic surgery pleurodesis): for recurrent or persistent leaks.

Complications

- Tension pneumothorax
- Recurrence
- Drain-related infection or bleeding
- Bronchopleural fistula
- Respiratory failure in individuals with limited reserve

Bibliography

British Thoracic Society. BTS pleural disease Guideline 2010. Thorax. 2010;65(Suppl 2):ii1–ii76.

Light RW. Pleural Diseases. 7th ed. Philadelphia: Wolters Kluwer; 2018.

Roberts DJ, Leigh-Smith S. Tension pneumothorax — time for a re-think? Emerg Med J. 2015;32(9):724–729.

59

Renal Replacement Therapy

Renal replacement therapy (RRT) encompasses techniques that artificially substitute the filtration and regulatory functions of the kidney when native renal function is severely compromised. It is utilised in both acute kidney injury (AKI) and chronic kidney disease (CKD) when conservative measures fail to sustain adequate homeostasis. In critical care, RRT is often used not only to remove solutes and water but also to stabilise the internal environment during systemic illness.

Pathophysiology and Indications

The kidneys normally regulate fluid and electrolyte balance, acid–base status, and remove metabolic waste products such as urea and creatinine. In AKI or advanced CKD, this ability is lost, leading to

- Uraemia that can lead to encephalopathy, pericarditis, and platelet dysfunction.
- Electrolyte imbalance that can lead to hyperkalaemia, hypocalcaemia, and hyperphosphataemia.
- Metabolic acidosis that leads to impaired cardiovascular and respiratory functions.
- Fluid overload that can lead to pulmonary oedema and refractory hypertension.

RRT is initiated when these derangements become life-threatening or resistant to medical therapy. The mnemonic AEIOU often remembers common clinical indications:

- Acidosis (severe, refractory metabolic acidosis).
- Electrolyte imbalance (notably hyperkalaemic > 6.5 mmol/L).
- Ingestions (toxin or drug removal, e.g. lithium, ethylene glycol).
- Overload (fluid overload unresponsive to diuretics).
- Uraemia (encephalopathy, pericarditis, bleeding).

Importantly, initiation is a clinical decision – based on trajectory and overall status rather than isolated creatinine or urea values.

Modalities of RRT

Intermittent Haemodialysis (IHD)

Intermittent haemodialysis (IHD) uses high blood and dialysate flow rates over 3–4 hours, usually three times weekly in chronic dialysis patients. It is highly effective at removing solutes and fluids but is often poorly tolerated in critically ill patients due to rapid shifts in volume and electrolytes, which can lead to hypotension or cerebral oedema.

Continuous Renal Replacement Therapy (CRRT)

In critical care, continuous therapies are preferred for unstable patients. They gradually remove solutes and fluid over 24 hours, ensuring haemodynamic stability and precise control of fluid balance. Subtypes include

- CVVH (continuous veno-venous haemofiltration): uses convective clearance with replacement fluid; effective for middle-molecule solutes.
- CVVHD (continuous veno-venous haemodialysis): a diffusive clearance method using dialysate; effective for removing small molecules such as urea.
- CVVHDF (continuous veno-venous haemodiafiltration): combines convection and diffusion; most commonly used in UK ICUs.
- SCUF (slow continuous ultrafiltration): designed for isolated fluid removal without solute clearance; useful in severe heart failure with fluid overload.

Hybrid Therapies

Techniques like sustained low-efficiency dialysis (SLED) combine aspects of both intermittent and continuous methods, running over 8–12 hours to ensure stability while using fewer resources.

Other Forms

- Peritoneal dialysis (PD): seldom employed in acute UK critical care but continues to be vital for long-term treatment in certain patients.
- Haemodiafiltration (HDF): an extension of haemodialysis, often employed in outpatient settings to improve middle molecule clearance.

Anticoagulation in RRT

Extracorporeal circuits are susceptible to clotting, especially in CRRT, where flows tend to be slower. Options include

- Regional citrate anticoagulation (RCA): favoured in many UK centres. Citrate chelates calcium in the circuit, preventing clotting, and is then metabolised in the liver, with calcium being replaced systemically. This provides a long filter lifespan with minimal risk of systemic bleeding.

- Unfractionated heparin: simple to use but increases systemic bleeding risk.
- No anticoagulation: sometimes used in patients with a high bleeding risk, although filter lifespan is shorter.

Vascular Access

RRT requires reliable venous access, typically via a double-lumen central venous catheter. The right internal jugular vein is preferred due to optimal flow and reduced complication risk. The femoral and subclavian veins serve as alternatives. Long-term RRT (CKD) necessitates arteriovenous fistulas or tunnelled lines.

Complications

Potential complications include

- Haemodynamic instability: hypotension during or after dialysis.
- Electrolyte derangements: hypokalaemia, hypophosphataemia, and hypocalcaemia with prolonged therapy.
- Bleeding: due to anticoagulation or platelet dysfunction.
- Infection: central line–associated bloodstream infection.
- Filter/circuit failure: clotting, kinking, or technical malfunction.
- Long-term effects: loss of nutrients through the filter (amino acids, micronutrients), and the risk of developing chronic dependence if renal recovery does not occur.

Monitoring and Supportive Care

Patients on RRT require close monitoring of

- Fluid balance and weight.
- Serum electrolytes, bicarbonate, phosphate, and calcium.
- Acid–base status.
- Haemodynamic status.
- Catheter site for infection.

Nutrition and drug dosing need to be adjusted, as many medications are removed by dialysis.

Prognosis and Outcomes

RRT in AKI is supportive – not curative – with outcomes depending on the underlying cause. Some patients recover renal function completely, while others develop CKD or require long-term dialysis. In critically ill patients, mortality remains high (40–60% in severe septic AKI). Early recognition of indications, careful selection of modalities, and integration with overall ICU management are essential for improving outcomes.

Bibliography

Bellomo R, Kellum JA, Ronco C. Acute renal failure — definition, outcome measures, animal models, fluid therapy and information technology needs. Crit Care. 2004;8:R204–R212.

Joannidis M, Oudemans-van Straaten HM. Clinical review: patency of the circuit in continuous renal replacement therapy. Crit Care. 2007;11:218.

James M, Ostermann M. KDIGO clinical practice guideline for acute kidney injury. Kidney Int Suppl. 2012;2:1–138.

National Institute for Health and Care Excellence (NICE). Acute kidney injury: prevention, detection and management (NG148). 2019.

Ronco C, Bellomo R, Kellum JA. Continuous renal replacement therapy: evolution in technology and current nomenclature. Kidney Int. 2018;94(6):1083–1089.

60

Pulmonary Oedema

Pulmonary oedema is a clinical condition characterised by the accumulation of excess fluid in the lung interstitium and alveoli, which hampers oxygen exchange. It is not a disease in itself but rather a sign of underlying cardiac or non-cardiac pathology. The presentation may be sudden and severe, as in flash pulmonary oedema, or more gradual in chronic heart failure. Prompt recognition and intervention are crucial, as severe cases can result in life-threatening respiratory failure.

Pathophysiology

Fluid movement through the pulmonary capillaries is controlled by Starling forces: hydrostatic pressure, oncotic pressure, and capillary permeability. In healthy conditions, these forces remain balanced to prevent fluid leakage into alveoli, with lymphatic drainage removing small amounts that escape.

- Cardiogenic pulmonary oedema occurs due to increased hydrostatic pressure in the pulmonary capillaries, usually caused by left ventricular systolic or diastolic dysfunction. As left atrial pressure increases, fluid is pushed from the capillaries into the interstitial space and alveoli. This fluid generally has low protein content.
- Non-cardiogenic pulmonary oedema results from increased capillary permeability, typically mediated by inflammation. In conditions like ARDS, sepsis, or inhalational injury, endothelial and epithelial damages permit the leakage of protein-rich fluid into the alveoli even in the absence of raised pressures.

In both mechanisms, alveolar flooding inactivates surfactant, reduces lung compliance, causes atelectasis, and impairs gas diffusion. The outcome is hypoxaemia, initially through ventilation–perfusion mismatch and later via shunt physiology.

Causes

Cardiogenic

- Left ventricular failure (e.g. post-MI, cardiomyopathy).
- Valvular disease (mitral stenosis, aortic stenosis/regurgitation).

- Arrhythmias (atrial fibrillation, tachyarrhythmias).
- Fluid overload (renal failure, aggressive IV fluid therapy).

Non-cardiogenic

- ARDS (sepsis, pancreatitis, trauma).
- Neurogenic (head injury, subarachnoid haemorrhage).
- High-altitude pulmonary oedema (HAPE).
- Drug/toxin exposure (opioids, salicylates, inhalational agents).
- Severe infections (viral pneumonia, malaria).

Clinical Features

The hallmark sign is acute dyspnoea. Other features include

- Orthopnoea and paroxysmal nocturnal dyspnoea.
- Pink, frothy sputum (alveolar flooding).
- Fine inspiratory crackles beginning at the bases, radiating upwards as severity increases.
- Tachypnoea, tachycardia, hypertension (early), or hypotension (late).
- Signs of underlying cardiac disease: gallop rhythm, raised JVP, peripheral oedema, and hepatomegaly.

Severe cases include distress, agitation, diaphoresis, and hypoxia, which can advance to cyanosis and respiratory failure.

Investigations

- ABG: type I respiratory failure (low PaO_2, normal or low $PaCO_2$); may progress to type II if severe fatigue occurs.
- Chest X-ray: cardiomegaly (common in cardiogenic cases), upper lobe diversion, Kerley B lines, perihilar 'bat-wing' shadowing, and pleural effusions.
- BNP/NT-proBNP: elevated in heart failure and assists in distinguishing cardiac from non-cardiac causes.
- ECG: ischaemia and arrhythmias.
- Echocardiography: used to evaluate ejection fraction and valvular disease.
- Bloods: U&Es, LFTs, troponin, CRP.

Management

Immediate management (ABCDE)

- Sit the patient upright and administer high-flow oxygen.
- IV furosemide to decrease preload.
- Glyceryl trinitrate (sublingual/IV) if BP permits, reducing preload and afterload.

- CPAP or BiPAP for ongoing hypoxia despite oxygen therapy.
- Inotropes (dobutamine, noradrenaline) in case of cardiogenic shock.
- Morphine is no longer routinely advised but may be considered for severe anxiety or distress.

Long-term management

- Optimise treatment for chronic heart failure: ACE inhibitors/ARBs, beta-blockers, MRAs, and SGLT2 inhibitors.
- Control risk factors: hypertension, arrhythmias, valvular disease, and ischaemia.
- Lifestyle: low-salt diet, fluid restriction, and daily weights.

Complications

- Severe respiratory failure needing intubation and mechanical ventilation.
- Cardiogenic shock.
- Recurrent hospitalisations due to decompensated heart failure.
- Progression to chronic heart failure accompanied by a reduced quality of life.

Bibliography

McMurray JJV, Pfeffer MA. Heart failure. Lancet. 2022;399(10334):181–194.

National Institute for Health and Care Excellence (NICE). Acute Heart Failure: Diagnosis and Management. NICE Guideline [NG106]; 2018.

Ponikowski P, Voors AA, Anker SD, et al. 2021 ESC Guidelines for the diagnosis and treatment of acute and chronic heart failure. Eur Heart J. 2021;42(36):3599–3726.

Ware LB, Matthay MA. Clinical practice. Acute pulmonary edema. N Engl J Med. 2005;353(26):2788–2796.

61

Sepsis

Sepsis is a life-threatening syndrome of organ dysfunction caused by a dysregulated host response to infection. It spans a spectrum from uncomplicated infection with systemic inflammation to septic shock, characterised by circulatory collapse, cellular dysfunction, and a high risk of death. Globally, sepsis is a significant cause of morbidity and mortality, especially among the very young, elderly, and immunocompromised.

Pathophysiology

Sepsis occurs when the body's immune response to infection becomes excessive and unbalanced. Pathogen-associated molecular patterns (PAMPs) and damage-associated molecular patterns (DAMPs) activate the innate immune system through toll-like receptors and other pathways. This causes a surge of pro-inflammatory cytokines (e.g. TNF-α, IL-1, IL-6) alongside anti-inflammatory mediators, leading to a 'cytokine storm'.

Widespread endothelial activation raises vascular permeability, resulting in capillary leak, tissue oedema, and hypovolaemia. At the same time, nitric oxide and prostaglandins cause vasodilation, lowering systemic vascular resistance and leading to distributive shock. The coagulation cascade is triggered, promoting microvascular thrombosis, while fibrinolysis is hindered, increasing the risk of disseminated intravascular coagulation (DIC).

At the cellular level, mitochondrial dysfunction decreases oxygen utilisation, worsening tissue hypoxia despite adequate delivery. Myocardial depression frequently occurs, reducing cardiac output further. These combined effects lead to multi-organ dysfunction, including acute kidney injury (AKI), acute respiratory distress syndrome (ARDS), encephalopathy, and hepatic failure.

Causes

Sepsis can originate from nearly any source of infection.

- Respiratory tract issues – pneumonia, aspiration, and viral superinfection.
- Urinary tract diseases – UTI, pyelonephritis, and urosepsis.

- Abdominal – peritonitis, perforation, cholangitis, and diverticulitis.
- Skin/soft tissue – cellulitis and necrotising fasciitis.
- Device-related – central venous catheters, urinary catheters, and prosthetic material.
- Central nervous system – meningitis and encephalitis.

Clinical Features

Sepsis may present subtly, especially in the elderly or individuals with immunosuppression. Common signs include

- Fever or hypothermia.
- Tachycardia and tachypnoea.
- Hypotension (systolic < 100 mmHg).
- Altered mental state (confusion, agitation, reduced GCS).
- Oliguria.
- Clinical evidence of infection (e.g. cough, flank pain, cellulitis).

Signs of severe sepsis/septic shock

- Mottled, cool peripheries
- Cyanosis
- Raised lactate and metabolic acidosis
- Multi-organ dysfunction (renal, respiratory, hepatic, coagulation)

Diagnosis

Sepsis is characterised by suspected or confirmed infection along with organ dysfunction.

qSOFA (quick Sequential Organ Failure Assessment)

- RR ≥ 22/min
- SBP ≤ 100 mmHg
- Altered mentation (GCS < 15)

A score of ≥2 signifies a higher risk of adverse outcome and requires prompt escalation.

Other supportive findings

- Lactate > 2 mmol/L
- AKI (rising creatinine, reduced urine output)
- Coagulopathy (prolonged PT/INR, low platelets)
- Deranged LFTs

Blood cultures, urine, sputum, or site-specific cultures should be taken before antibiotics, but without delaying treatment.

Management

Prompt recognition and early intervention are crucial, preferably within the first hour of suspicion.

Sepsis six (UK model)

1) Give oxygen to maintain saturations.
2) Take blood cultures.
3) Administer IV antibiotics (broad-spectrum, within 1 hour).
4) Give IV fluids (e.g. crystalloids).
5) Check lactate.
6) Monitor urine output.

Further measures might encompass

- Source control (e.g. drain abscess, remove infected line).
- Use vasopressors (norepinephrine) if hypotension persists after fluids.
- ICU referral for organ support (ventilation, Renal Replacement Therapy (RRT)).
- Glycaemic control, stress ulcer prophylaxis, and thromboprophylaxis.

Complications

- Septic shock with refractory hypotension
- ARDS
- AKI
- DIC
- Multi-organ failure
- High mortality (30–50% in septic shock)

Bibliography

NICE. Sepsis: Recognition, Diagnosis and Early Management [NG51]. National Institute for Health and Care Excellence; 2016.

Rhodes A, Evans LE, Alhazzani W, et al. Surviving sepsis campaign: international guidelines for management of sepsis and septic shock: 2016. Intensive Care Med. 2017;43:304–377.

Singer M, Deutschman CS, Seymour CW, et al. The third international consensus definitions for sepsis and septic shock (sepsis-3). JAMA. 2016;315(8):801–810.

62

Spinal Cord Injury

Spinal cord injury (SCI) is damage to the spinal cord or cauda equina that causes motor, sensory, and autonomic dysfunction below the level of the lesion. It most commonly results from trauma, such as road traffic collisions, falls, sporting injuries, or penetrating trauma, but can also be caused by non-traumatic factors including tumours, infection, vascular malformations, and ischaemia. SCI has high morbidity and mortality. Early recognition, appropriate resuscitation, and multidisciplinary care are vital to improve outcomes and minimise long-term disability.

Pathophysiology

The spinal cord extends from the foramen magnum to the L1–L2 vertebral level, where it tapers into the conus medullaris and cauda equina. Vertebrae, meninges, cerebrospinal fluid, and surrounding musculature protect it. Functionally, it is organised into ascending and descending tracts.

- Corticospinal tracts: motor control.
- Spinothalamic tracts: pain and temperature sensation.
- Dorsal columns: proprioception, vibration, and delicate touch.

This anatomical organisation underpins the varied clinical syndromes that can occur with SCI.

Primary Injury

The initial injury may involve fracture, dislocation, compression, laceration, or penetrating trauma, leading to disruption of axons, haemorrhage, and immediate loss of neural tissue.

Secondary Injury

Secondary injury develops over minutes to weeks and greatly influences neurological deterioration. Mechanisms include

- Ischaemia and hypoperfusion resulting from microvascular damage.
- Inflammatory cascade characterised by infiltration of neutrophils and macrophages releasing cytokines.

- Excitotoxicity, especially glutamate-mediated neuronal death.
- Oxidative stress and free radical production damage membranes and DNA.
- Oedema and increased intrathecal pressure, which worsen cord hypoxia.

Together, these processes form a cycle of ongoing tissue loss, scarring, and reduced regeneration.

Classification

- By level
  - Tetraplegia: injury at C1–T1 that impacts all four limbs.
  - Paraplegia: injury between T2 and L1, affecting the trunk and lower limbs.
- By completeness (American Spinal Injury Association Impairment Scale, AIS):
  - A: Complete (no sensory or motor function preserved in sacral segments).
  - B–D: Incomplete, with varying preservation of function.
  - E: Normal.

Incomplete Syndromes

Anterior cord syndrome: loss of motor function, pain, and temperature sensation below the lesion; proprioception remains intact.

Central cord syndrome: greater weakness in the upper limbs compared to the lower; commonly occurs after cervical hyperextension.

Brown-Séquard syndrome: ipsilateral loss of motor function and proprioception with contralateral loss of pain and temperature.

Cauda equina syndrome: features of lower motor neuron damage with saddle anaesthesia, urinary retention, and flaccid paralysis – a neurosurgical emergency.

Assessment

All trauma patients should be considered to have a spinal injury until it is ruled out. Initial management follows ABCDE with spinal precautions:

- Rigid collar, head blocks, and spinal board or vacuum mattress.
- High cervical injuries pose a risk of diaphragmatic paralysis (C3–C5); remain vigilant for airway compromise.
- Neurogenic shock (bradycardia, hypotension, warm peripheries) can occur in cervical or upper thoracic lesions.

A comprehensive neurological examination should be recorded on the American Spinal Injury Association (ASIA)/ International Standards for Neurological Classifications of Spinal Cord Injury (ISNSCI) chart, assessing

- Motor and sensory levels.
- Sacral sparing (anal tone, voluntary contraction, perianal sensation).
- Priapism, which can signify complete SCI.

Investigations

- CT spine: first-line investigation for fractures or instability.
- MRI: crucial for evaluating cord compression, haemorrhage, or oedema.
- Bloods: FBC, U&E, coagulation profile, and lactate.

Acute Management

- Airway and breathing: consider early intubation in cases of high cervical injury or declining GCS.
- Circulation: keep mean arterial pressure above 85–90 mmHg using vasopressors (noradrenaline preferred); fluids alone are insufficient in neurogenic shock.
- Maintain spinal alignment consistently.
- Surgery: early decompression and stabilisation where necessary.
- Steroids: high-dose methylprednisolone is no longer routinely recommended because of limited benefit and significant risks.
- Bladder management: catheterisation to prevent retention.

Complications

- Respiratory failure resulting from cervical injuries.
- Neurogenic bladder and bowel dysfunction.
- Pressure ulcers and recurring infections.
- Venous thromboembolism – necessitates early thromboprophylaxis.
- Spasticity and chronic pain syndromes.
- Autonomic dysreflexia (in lesions above T6): sudden rise in blood pressure, headache, and flushing, triggered by bladder or bowel irritation.
- Psychological sequelae, such as depression, anxiety, and Post Traumatic Stress Disorder (PTSD).

63

Rehabilitation and Long-Term Care

Multidisciplinary rehabilitation is essential and includes physiotherapy, occupational therapy, speech and language therapy, psychology, and specialised nursing. Goals focus on

- Maximising independence and mobility.
- Preventing complications.
- Supporting community reintegration, vocational rehabilitation, and long-term bladder, bowel, and sexual health management.

Long-term care also includes pain management, spasticity control, and routine screening for complications such as osteoporosis and renal impairment.

Bibliography

Ahuja CS, Wilson JR, Nori S, et al. Traumatic spinal cord injury. Nat Rev Dis Primers. 2017;3:17018.

Badhiwala JH, Wilson JR, Fehlings MG. Global burden of traumatic brain and spinal cord injury. Lancet Neurol. 2019;18(1):24–25.

Furlan JC, Noonan V, Cadotte DW, Fehlings MG. Timing of decompressive surgery of spinal cord after traumatic spinal cord injury: a systematic review of the literature. Neurosurg Focus. 2008;25(5):E2.

National Institute for Health and Care Excellence (NICE). Spinal Injury: Assessment and Initial Management. NICE guideline [NG41]; 2016.

64

Status Epilepticus

Status epilepticus (SE) is a neurological emergency characterised by a seizure lasting longer than 5 minutes or recurrent seizures without full recovery of consciousness in between. It can cause neuronal damage, systemic complications, and death if not treated quickly.

Pathophysiology

Normal seizures terminate through intrinsic inhibitory mechanisms involving GABAergic pathways. In SE, persistent excitation or failure of inhibition leads to prolonged electrical activity. Over time, this results in receptor trafficking (Gamma-aminobutyric (GABA) receptor internalisation and N-methyl-D-aspartate (NMDA) receptor upregulation), making seizures harder to treat the longer they persist continue.

Prolonged seizures increase metabolic demand, reduce cerebral perfusion, and raise intracranial pressure, which can cause neuronal death. Systemically, SE may lead to hypoxia, lactic acidosis, rhabdomyolysis, hyperthermia, and cardiac arrhythmias.

Causes

- Epilepsy (non-compliance, drug withdrawal)
- Structural lesions (stroke, tumour, trauma)
- Infection (meningitis, encephalitis)
- Metabolic (hypoglycaemia, hyponatraemia, uraemia)
- Alcohol/drug withdrawal
- Toxins or overdose (e.g. Tricyclic antidepressants (TCAs), Isoniazid (INH))
- Idiopathic

Clinical Presentation

- Generalised convulsions (tonic–clonic movements).
- Focal seizures with impaired awareness.

- Non-convulsive SE: altered consciousness, confusion, and twitching.
- Prolonged postictal state.

Be vigilant for subtle signs in intubated or sedated patients – status may continue without visible seizure activity.

Initial Management Approach

Airway, breathing, and circulation are the priorities – ensure oxygenation and secure IV access. Check bedside glucose and treat hypoglycaemia if present.

Simultaneously

- Administer benzodiazepines.
- Start second-line antiepileptic if seizures last more than 10 minutes.
- Escalate to critical care and anaesthetic support if refractory.

Drug Management Table

Step	Timeframe	Medication	Dose	Route	Notes
1st line	0 5 min	Lorazepam	4 mg	IV	Preferred IV benzo, may repeat once after 10–15 min
		Diazepam	10 mg	IV	Shorter acting, may need repeating sooner
		Midazolam (if no IV)	10 mg (5 mg if elderly/frail)	Buccal/IM	Common in pre-hospital settings
2nd Line	5–20 min	Levetiracetam	20–60 mg/kg (max 4.5 g)	IV over 5–10 min	Often first-line second agent due to safety
		Phenytoin	20 mg/kg	IV over 30 min	Avoid if already on it; risk of arrhythmia; ECG monitoring needed
		Sodium valproate	20–30 mg/kg (max 3 g)	IV over 15 min	Avoid in young females or hepatic disease
3rd line	20–40+ min	Propofol/ midazolam infusion/ thiopentone	Titrated to EEG burst suppression	IV infusion	Requires intubation and ICU management (refractory SE)

Investigations

- Capillary glucose (rule out hypoglycaemia immediately).
- Bloods: FBC, U&Es, calcium, magnesium, LFTs, toxicology screen, and drug levels (e.g. phenytoin, Anti-epileptic drug (AEDs)).
- ABG (for lactate, acidosis, oxygenation).
- CT/MRI brain if new or focal signs.
- EEG to identify non-convulsive SE or subtle seizures.

Complications

- Hypoxia and aspiration pneumonia
- Acidosis and hyperkalaemia
- Rhabdomyolysis and AKI
- Cerebral oedema and permanent brain injury
- Multi-organ failure and death

Bibliography

Brophy GM, Bell R, Claassen J, et al. Guidelines for the evaluation and management of status epilepticus. Neurocrit Care. 2012;17(1):3–23.

National Institute for Health and Care Excellence (NICE). Epilepsies: Diagnosis and Management. NICE Guideline NG217; 2022.

Shorvon S, Ferlisi M. The treatment of super-refractory status epilepticus: a critical review of available therapies and a clinical treatment protocol. Brain. 2011;134(10):2802–2818.

Trinka E, Cock H, Hesdorffer D, et al. A definition and classification of status epilepticus—Report of the ILAE Task Force on Classification of Status Epilepticus. Epilepsia. 2015;56(10):1515–1523.

65

Shock Overview

Shock is a life-threatening condition of circulatory failure that results in insufficient tissue perfusion and oxygen delivery. It causes cellular hypoxia, metabolic disturbances, and ultimately multi-organ failure if not treated promptly. Shock is categorised into four main types: hypovolaemic, cardiogenic, distributive, and obstructive. Early detection and intervention are essential for better outcomes.

Pathophysiology

Shock happens when oxygen delivery (DO_2) cannot satisfy tissue oxygen demand (VO_2). Mechanisms include

- Inadequate circulating volume (hypovolaemia).
- Pump failure (cardiogenic).
- Maldistribution of blood flow (distributive).
- Physical obstruction to cardiac output (obstructive).

Common features across all types

- Cellular shift to anaerobic metabolism leads to lactate accumulation.
- Mitochondrial dysfunction and impaired ATP synthesis.
- Prolonged systemic inflammatory response.
- Progression to multi-organ failure if left untreated.

Types of Shock

Type	Common Causes	Key Features	Management Principles
Hypovolaemic	Haemorrhage (trauma, GI bleed), dehydration, and burns	Tachycardia, hypotension, cool peripheries, and collapsed neck veins	Volume replacement (blood, crystalloids) and control bleeding/source
Cardiogenic	MI, arrhythmia, myocarditis, and cardiomyopathy	Hypotension, raised JVP, pulmonary oedema, and cool peripheries	Inotropes (dobutamine), vasopressors, revascularisation, and treat arrhythmias
Distributive	Sepsis, anaphylaxis, and spinal/ neurogenic	Warm peripheries early (sepsis), low Systemic vascular resistance (SVR), bounding pulse; anaphylaxis: urticaria and airway swelling	Vasopressors (noradrenaline first-line in sepsis), IV fluids, treat cause (antibiotics, adrenaline in anaphylaxis)
Obstructive	PE, cardiac tamponade, and tension pneumothorax	Sudden collapse, raised JVP, pulsus paradoxus, and absent breath sounds (pneumothorax)	Relieve obstruction (thrombolysis, pericardiocentesis, needle decompression)

Clinical Features

- Early signs: tachycardia, tachypnoea, anxiety, and reduced urine output.
- Late signs: hypotension, altered mental state, mottled and cool peripheries, and lactic acidosis.
- Indicators of poor perfusion: low urine output (<0.5 mL/kg/hr), high lactate levels, narrow pulse pressure (hypovolaemia or cardiogenic), or wide pulse pressure (distributive).

Investigations

- Bedside: ECG, capillary glucose, arterial blood gas (ABG) (look for lactate, metabolic acidosis).
- Laboratory tests: full blood count (FBC), U&Es, coagulation profile, liver function tests (LFTs), troponin, and blood cultures.
- Imaging
  - CXR (pneumothorax, pulmonary oedema)
  - Echocardiography (tamponade, cardiac function, valve disease)
  - CT (PE, intra-abdominal bleed, sepsis source)

Management

Initial resuscitation follows an ABCDE approach with concurrent diagnosis and treatment.

- Airway and breathing: provide oxygen; consider intubation if breathing fails.
- Circulation:
  - Establish IV/IO access, and monitor ECG, BP, SpO_2, and urine output.
  - Fluid resuscitation in hypovolaemia or distributive shock.
  - Early administration of vasopressors in distributive and cardiogenic shock (noradrenaline as first-line in sepsis, adrenaline in anaphylaxis).
  - Inotropes (dobutamine, milrinone) if contractility is impaired.
  - Use blood products if haemorrhage occurs, guided by the massive transfusion protocol.
- Definitive management: consistently address the underlying cause (e.g. source control in sepsis, PCI in MI, decompression in tamponade).
- Monitoring: arterial line for invasive blood pressure, central access for vasopressors, serial lactate, and urine output.

Prognosis

Prognosis depends on the type of shock, the speed of recognition, and the reversal of the underlying cause. Mortality remains high in septic and cardiogenic shock despite advances in treatment. Early goal-directed resuscitation, protocolised care (e.g. sepsis bundles), and a multidisciplinary team improve survival.

Bibliography

Cecconi M, De Backer D, Antonelli M, et al. Consensus on circulatory shock and hemodynamic monitoring. Intensive Care Med. 2014;40(12):1795–1815.

NICE. Intravenous fluid therapy in adults in hospital (CG174). 2023 update.

Resuscitation Council UK. ALS guidelines: shock and peri-arrest arrhythmias. 2021.

Singer M, Deutschman CS, Seymour CW, et al. The third international consensus definitions for sepsis and septic shock (sepsis-3). JAMA. 2016;315(8):801–810.

66

Stroke

Stroke is a leading cause of illness and death in the United Kingdom and worldwide. It occurs when blood flow to a part of the brain is interrupted, resulting in ischaemia, infarction, and neurological issues. Strokes are primarily classified as ischaemic (85%) or haemorrhagic (15%). Early detection and treatment are vital for reducing brain damage and improving functional recovery.

Pathophysiology

An ischaemic stroke occurs when blood flow to a part of the brain is blocked, depriving neurons of oxygen and nutrients. This is the most common form of stroke, accounting for the majority of cases in the United Kingdom. The underlying mechanisms vary. Thrombotic occlusion often results from atherosclerotic disease in large vessels such as the internal carotid artery or middle cerebral artery. Embolic events are another major cause and often arise from atrial fibrillation, which encourages clot formation in the left atrium. These emboli can also come from mural thrombus following a recent myocardial infarction or from valvular heart disease, especially in the presence of prosthetic valves or infective endocarditis. A further category includes small vessel or lacunar infarcts, which are strongly linked to chronic hypertension and diabetes. Although small in size, lacunar infarcts can cause significant neurological deficits depending on their location.

The pathophysiological cascade following cerebral ischaemia is well established. When perfusion drops below a critical threshold, neuronal ATP production ceases, leading to dysfunction of energy-dependent ion pumps. Sodium and calcium ions build up within cells, causing cytotoxic oedema. Excess intracellular calcium triggers the release of excitatory neurotransmitters such as glutamate, which worsens injury through excitotoxicity. This process quickly forms an infarct core of irreversibly damaged tissue. Surrounding this is the penumbra, an area of hypo-perfused but still viable brain tissue. The penumbra remains at risk of infarction but can potentially be saved if timely reperfusion therapy, such as thrombolysis or mechanical thrombectomy, is provided. This concept emphasises the importance of rapid recognition and treatment of ischaemic stroke.

Haemorrhagic stroke is a different but equally devastating condition. It occurs when a cerebral blood vessel ruptures, leading to bleeding within or around the brain. Intracerebral haemorrhage is most often caused by chronic hypertension, which weakens small penetrating arteries, or cerebral amyloid angiopathy, where abnormal amyloid deposits make vessels fragile. The accumulation of blood within brain tissue causes direct neuronal injury, mass effect from the expanding haematoma, and increased intracranial pressure. These processes can result in rapid neurological deterioration and herniation if left untreated.

Clinical Features

Stroke symptoms usually appear suddenly and indicate the affected vascular area.

Territory	Typical Deficits
Middle cerebral artery (MCA)	Contralateral hemiparesis (face/arm > leg), aphasia (dominant hemisphere), and neglect (non-dominant)
Anterior cerebral artery (ACA)	Contralateral leg weakness, behavioural changes, and urinary incontinence
Posterior cerebral artery (PCA)	Visual field deficits (homonymous hemianopia) and memory impairment
Brainstem	Cranial nerve palsies, crossed findings (ipsilateral face + contralateral body weakness), and respiratory compromise
Cerebellar	Ataxia, dysarthria, vertigo, and nystagmus

Other features may include dysphagia, altered consciousness, seizures, or gaze deviation. In elderly or frail patients, presentations may be more subtle.

Diagnosis

The diagnosis is primarily clinical, supported by imaging and tests to identify the type and cause of stroke.

- CT Head (non-contrast): first line, to exclude haemorrhage and detect ischaemia (may be normal in early hours).
- CT angiography (CTA): detects large vessel occlusion, guiding thrombectomy.
- CT perfusion/MRI DWI: utilised in select centres to delineate infarct core and penumbra.
- Blood tests: glucose (to rule out hypoglycaemia), FBC, U&E, clotting, and lipids.
- ECG/echocardiography: to identify atrial fibrillation or other cardioembolic sources.

Management

Immediate priorities

- Administer the ABCDE approach with oxygen if hypoxic.
- Rapid glucose test to exclude mimics.
- Urgent referral to a hyperacute stroke unit.

Ischaemic stroke

- Thrombolysis: IV alteplase administered within 4.5 hours of symptom onset (NICE). Contraindications include recent surgery, bleeding risk, or very high blood pressure.
- Mechanical thrombectomy: for large vessel occlusion within 6 hours, and in selected cases up to 24 hours, guided by advanced imaging.
- Antiplatelet therapy: Aspirin 300 mg, initiated after haemorrhage has been ruled out.
- Secondary prevention: long-term antiplatelets (e.g. clopidogrel), anticoagulation for AF, high-intensity statins, and BP and diabetes management.
- Conduct swallow assessment within 4 hours of admission; provide nutritional support as indicated.

Haemorrhagic stroke

- Urgent neurosurgical referral: for haematoma evacuation, decompression, or aneurysm repair (clipping/coiling).
- Blood pressure control: target SBP < 140–160 mmHg (NICE).
- Reverse anticoagulation using PCC, vitamin K, or specific reversal agents.
- ICP monitoring and management in neurocritical care.

Complications

- Neurological: cerebral oedema, seizures, and recurrent stroke.
- Respiratory conditions: aspiration pneumonia and respiratory failure.
- Cardiovascular: arrhythmias, cardiac ischaemia, and venous thromboembolism.
- Psychological: depression, cognitive impairment, anxiety, and post-stroke fatigue.

Rehabilitation and Secondary Prevention

Stroke recovery requires a multidisciplinary approach involving physiotherapists, occupational therapists, speech and language therapists, psychologists, and stroke nurses. Early mobilisation, intensive therapy, and family support enhance outcomes. Most recovery occurs within the first 3–6 months, but long-term rehabilitation remains essential.

Secondary prevention strategies comprise

- Antiplatelets or anticoagulants (depending on the cause).
- Management of blood pressure, glucose, and lipids.

- Lifestyle modifications such as quitting smoking, healthy diet, and regular exercise.
- Education and support for patients and carers.

Bibliography

European Stroke Organisation (ESO). Guidelines on stroke management. 2021.

National Institute for Health and Care Excellence (NICE). Stroke and Transient Ischaemic Attack in Over 16s: Diagnosis and Initial Management. NICE Guideline [NG128]; 2019.

Powers WJ, Rabinstein AA, Ackerson T, et al. Guidelines for the early management of acute ischemic stroke. Stroke. 2018;49(3):e46–e110.

Royal College of Physicians. National clinical guideline for stroke. 2023.

Stroke Association. State of the nation: stroke statistics. 2023.

67

Tracheostomies

A tracheostomy is a surgically created opening in the front of the trachea that provides direct access to the airway. A tracheostomy tube is inserted into this opening to bypass the upper airway, assist with mechanical ventilation, enable the clearance of secretions, and, in some cases, offer long-term airway protection. Tracheostomies may be temporary or permanent and can be performed via

- Surgical tracheostomy – typically performed in theatre, often chosen when anatomy is complicated or urgent access is needed.
- Percutaneous tracheostomy – commonly performed at the bedside in critical care, less invasive and increasingly becoming the standard approach for ventilated patients.

Indications

- Prolonged mechanical ventilation (usually over 7–10 days).
- Upper airway obstruction (tumour, trauma, swelling, infection).
- Facilitation of secretion management (e.g. neuromuscular disease, bulbar dysfunction).
- Airway protection for patients with impaired consciousness or reduced airway reflexes.

Types of Tracheostomy Tubes

- Cuffed vs. uncuffed
  - Cuffed: permits positive pressure ventilation and reduces aspiration risk.
  - Uncuffed: used when airway protection is not required, facilitating easier speech and swallowing.
- Fenestrated vs. non-fenestrated
  - Fenestrated: having an opening that permits airflow through the vocal cords, assisting phonation.
- Inner cannula
  - Removable inner tubes make cleaning easier and allow quick replacement if blocked.

- Speaking valves (e.g. Passy-Muir)
  - One-way valves that allow speech during exhalation; require cuff deflation and a patent upper airway.

Routine Care

- Humidification – essential, since natural humidification is bypassed.
- Suctioning – performed using sterile technique when secretions are excessive or audible; should not be done routinely.
- Stoma care – daily cleaning with sterile saline, and monitoring for infection or skin breakdown.
- Cuff pressure monitoring should be checked regularly; keep below 25 cmH_2O to prevent mucosal damage.
- Tube changes – in line with local policy; ENT or critical care typically conduct the initial change.

Emergency Complications

Problem	Signs	Action
Tube dislodgement	Sudden respiratory distress and visible stoma	Call for help, apply oxygen to the stoma and mouth, and attempt reinsertion or oral intubation
Blockage	Increased work of breathing, inability to suction	Remove the inner cannula or replace the tube
Bleeding	Fresh bleeding and possible sentinel bleed	Suspect tracheo-innominate fistula; apply pressure, urgent ENT/vascular input
Subcutaneous emphysema	Swelling, crepitus around the stoma	May indicate false passage or trauma; seek urgent review

Tip: Always keep a tracheostomy emergency kit within easy reach of the patient's bedside.

Weaning and Decannulation

Weaning starts when the patient can protect their airway, handle secretions, and sustain spontaneous breathing. Steps include

1) Reducing the size of the tracheostomy tube.
2) Cuff deflation and speaking valve or capping trials.
3) Decannulation was once tolerated safely.

This process is typically led by critical care or ENT, with vital input from speech and language therapists, physiotherapists, and nursing staff.

Bibliography

Durbin CG. Tracheostomy: why, when, and how? Respir Care. 2010;55(8):1056–1068.

Intensive Care Society. Standards for the Care of Adult Patients with a Temporary Tracheostomy. London: ICS; 2020.

St John RE, Malen JF. Management of tracheostomies in critical care. Crit Care Nurse. 2004;24(5):26–37.

McGrath BA, Wallace S, Lynch J, Wilson M, Nicholson L, Dunwoody L. The UK National Tracheostomy Safety Project: developing the safety culture in airway management. Br J Anaesth. 2012;109(1):88–91.

National Tracheostomy Safety Project. n.d. NTSP guidelines and resources. https://www.tracheostomy.org.uk (Accessed 2025).

68

Transplant Overview

Organ transplantation involves replacing a diseased or failing organ with a healthy one from a donor. It is often life-saving or life-enhancing and is now regularly performed across major organ systems, including the kidney, liver, heart, lung, pancreas, and intestine. Donors may be living (e.g. kidney, liver lobe) or deceased. Details about organ donation processes are provided in a separate chapter.

Types of Transplantation

- Solid organ transplant
  - Kidney: the most common cause; related to end-stage renal disease.
  - Liver: indicated in cirrhosis, acute liver failure, or metabolic disease.
  - Heart: for advanced heart failure unresponsive to medical therapy.
  - Lung: for end-stage lung disease (e.g. COPD, cystic fibrosis).
  - Pancreas: typically combined with kidney transplantation in cases of diabetes.
  - Intestine: rare; utilised in cases of intestinal failure or short bowel syndrome.
- Haematopoietic stem cell transplant (HSCT): used for malignancies such as leukaemia or aplastic anaemia. Unlike solid organ transplants, it involves immune reconstitution and carries specific risks (e.g. graft-versus-host disease).

Matching and Immunology

Successful transplantation depends on immune compatibility between donor and recipient.

- ABO blood group compatibility.
- HLA (human leukocyte antigen) matching – especially crucial in kidney transplantation.
- Cross-matching ensures that the recipient has no pre-existing antibodies against the donor.

Modern immunomodulatory protocols sometimes allow ABO-incompatible or sensitised transplants through desensitisation strategies.

Immunosuppression

Recipients need lifelong immunosuppression to avoid rejection. Regimens usually consist of

- Induction therapy: strong immunosuppression administered at the time of transplant (e.g. basiliximab, antithymocyte globulin).
- Maintenance therapy
  - Calcineurin inhibitors (tacrolimus, cyclosporin)
  - Antiproliferative agents (mycophenolate mofetil)
  - Corticosteroids (prednisolone)

The balance is preventing rejection while minimising infection, malignancy, and drug toxicity.

Types of Rejection

- Hyperacute rejection: immediate; caused by pre-formed antibodies. Rare with modern cross-matching.
- Acute rejection: occurs days to weeks after transplant; typically T-cell mediated. May manifest as graft dysfunction.
- Chronic rejection: gradual graft failure over months or years, often irreversible.

Diagnosis relies on clinical features, laboratory findings, imaging, and biopsy.

Complications

Category	Examples
Infection	Opportunistic infections (CMV, EBV, *Pneumocystis*) and reactivation (e.g. TB, herpes)
Malignancy	Post-transplant lymphoproliferative disorder (PTLD) and skin cancers
Graft dysfunction	Rejection, drug toxicity, and recurrence of the original disease
Drug side effects	Nephrotoxicity (tacrolimus), hyperglycaemia, hypertension, and dyslipidaemia

Close specialist follow-up is essential for early detection of complications.

Ethics and Donor Considerations

In the United Kingdom, the Human Tissue Act regulates deceased donation and the opt-out system, known as 'deemed consent', although families are still consulted. Organs are allocated based on urgency, compatibility, and waiting time.

Living donation (usually kidney or liver lobe) requires a comprehensive medical, psychosocial, and legal assessment, especially in unrelated donors.

Conclusion

Transplant medicine is a complex, multidisciplinary field. For general hospital clinicians, priorities include recognising early complications, understanding common immunosuppressive regimens, avoiding harm (e.g. nephrotoxic drugs, uncontrolled infections), and involving specialist teams promptly. With appropriate care, transplant recipients can achieve excellent long-term outcomes.

Bibliography

British Transplantation Society. Guidelines for Transplantation. BTS; 2022.

Human Tissue Authority. Code of Practice F: Donation of Solid Organs and Tissue for Transplantation. London: HTA; 2020.

KDIGO Transplant Work Group. KDIGO clinical practice guideline for the care of kidney transplant recipients. Kidney Int Suppl. 2009;113:S1–S155.

NHS Blood and Transplant. Organ Donation and Transplantation in the UK. NHSBT; 2023.

69

Trauma Resuscitation

Trauma is a leading cause of death and disability worldwide, particularly affecting young adults. In the United Kingdom, trauma remains a major public health issue, resulting in thousands of deaths each year and significantly contributing to long-term health problems. Globally, trauma ranks as the fourth leading cause of death across all age groups and is the primary cause of death for those under 40. Most fatalities are due to road traffic accidents, falls, interpersonal violence, and workplace incidents.

Over the past decade, the development of trauma networks within the NHS has significantly improved outcomes, ensuring that seriously injured patients are promptly transferred to major trauma centres where multidisciplinary expertise and advanced imaging are readily available. For critical care practitioners, trauma remains one of the most challenging fields, requiring rapid assessment, prioritisation, and coordination of interventions under intense time constraints.

Resuscitation of the major trauma patient follows a systematic approach. The principles are consistent: life-threatening issues are identified and managed in order of urgency, guided by the Advanced Trauma Life Support (ATLS) framework. The process begins with the primary survey (ABCDE), followed by resuscitation, additional investigations, and a secondary survey to ensure a thorough injury assessment.

Primary Survey (ABCDE Approach)

The primary survey is the foundation of trauma resuscitation, designed to detect and address immediate threats to life. Each step must be carried out systematically, with interventions implemented promptly as issues are identified.

Airway with Cervical Spine Protection

The priority is to secure a patent airway while simultaneously protecting the cervical spine in any patient with potential head, neck, or high-energy injury. Signs of airway compromise include stridor, gurgling, hoarseness, and paradoxical chest movements.

- Basic manoeuvres (jaw thrust, suction, airway adjuncts such as oropharyngeal or nasopharyngeal airways) should be attempted initially.

- Definitive airway management: endotracheal intubation is indicated for patients with reduced consciousness (Glasgow Coma Scale [GCS] ≤ 8), airway obstruction, or a predicted clinical course requiring ventilation. Rapid sequence induction (RSI) with manual in-line stabilisation remains the standard.
- A surgical airway (needle cricothyroidotomy or surgical cricothyroidotomy) may be necessary if intubation proves impossible.

Protection of the cervical spine is compulsory until a radiological investigation rules out injury. This includes a rigid collar, blocks, and straps to limit movement.

Breathing

Once the airway is secured, the next step is to evaluate ventilation and oxygenation. Immediately recognise and manage life-threatening thoracic injuries, which include

- Tension pneumothorax – requires immediate needle decompression followed by chest drain insertion.
- Open pneumothorax – managed with an occlusive dressing secured on three sides, then chest drain.
- Massive haemothorax – insert a large-bore chest drain, provide fluid and blood resuscitation, and arrange early surgical referral.
- Flail chest with respiratory compromise – requires analgesia, oxygen support, and often intubation with positive pressure ventilation.

All trauma patients should receive high-flow oxygen initially, with monitoring through pulse oximetry and arterial blood gas analysis when feasible.

Circulation with Haemorrhage Control

Uncontrolled haemorrhage is the foremost preventable cause of death in trauma. Swift identification and control of bleeding are therefore vital.

- Control external bleeding using direct pressure, haemostatic dressings, and tourniquets if needed.
- IV/IO access: two large-bore IV cannulas should be inserted, or intraosseous access if IV access is not possible.
- Fluid resuscitation: in patients in shock, balanced transfusion (red cells, plasma, platelets) is preferred over crystalloid. Current UK major haemorrhage protocols recommend a 1:1:1 ratio.
- Permissive hypotension: target systolic BP of 80–90 mmHg (MAP ~65 mmHg) in uncontrolled haemorrhage until definitive control is achieved, except in traumatic brain injury (TBI), where higher pressures are required.

Assessment tools include blood pressure, heart rate, capillary refill, and mental status. Focused Assessment with Sonography for Trauma (FAST) can quickly detect intraperitoneal fluid; however, a negative scan does not rule out the possibility of bleeding.

Disability (Neurological Status)

A quick neurological assessment is crucial in trauma.

- The GCS is documented at the scene and upon arrival.
- Pupillary size, symmetry, and reactivity offer clues to raised ICP or focal lesions.
- Hypoglycaemia should be ruled out as a reversible cause of impaired consciousness.

Any deterioration in neurological status requires urgent investigation and possible intervention (airway management, CT head, neurosurgical referral).

Exposure and Environment

The patient must be fully exposed to identify hidden injuries, while taking care to prevent hypothermia – part of the 'lethal triad' (hypothermia, coagulopathy, acidosis) that worsens outcomes in trauma.

- Use warm blankets, fluid warmers, and heated environments where possible.
- Inspect for lacerations, abrasions, deformities, and seatbelt or handlebar marks that may suggest underlying injury.

Secondary Survey

Once immediate life-threatening issues have been managed and resuscitation has begun, attention shifts to the secondary survey. This is a structured head-to-toe assessment designed to find all injuries, including those not immediately visible during the primary survey.

Principles

- The secondary survey is only performed once the patient is stabilised and ongoing resuscitation measures are in place.
- It includes a full history (AMPLE: Allergies, Medications, Past medical history, Last meal, Events leading up to trauma) and a systematic examination from head to toe.
- Adjunct investigations are included at this stage, such as imaging, laboratory tests, and specialist referrals.

Key Components

- Head and face: examine for scalp lacerations, facial fractures, orbital injuries, and cerebrospinal fluid leaks.
- Neck: examine for penetrating trauma, tracheal deviation, jugular venous distension, or subcutaneous emphysema.
- Chest: reassess breathing, auscultate for breath sounds, palpate for crepitus or instability, and repeat imaging if condition worsens.
- Abdomen: palpate for tenderness, distension, or rigidity. FAST or diagnostic peritoneal aspirate may guide decision-making.
- Pelvis: assess stability with gentle pressure; unstable pelvises should be stabilised immediately using a pelvic binder.
- Limbs: evaluate for deformities, fractures, and neurovascular compromise.
- Back and spine: log-roll with spinal precautions to check for penetrating injury, bruising, or step deformity.

Imaging and Adjuncts

- FAST scan: bedside ultrasound to detect intraperitoneal or pericardial fluid.
- Chest and pelvic radiographs: quick screening for fractures and thoracic injury.
- CT pan-scan: increasingly utilised in major trauma centres to deliver rapid, comprehensive imaging of the head, chest, abdomen, and pelvis in haemodynamically stable patients.

The secondary survey should be repeated regularly, as injuries can develop or become apparent later in the clinical course.

Major Haemorrhage and Shock

Importance

Uncontrolled bleeding is the leading preventable cause of trauma death. Up to one-third of major trauma patients present with significant haemorrhage, and once haemorrhagic shock occurs, outcomes are greatly affected by the speed of diagnosis and the start of damage control resuscitation (DCR).

Classification of Shock in Trauma

Shock is broadly divided into

- Hypovolaemic (haemorrhagic) – most common in trauma, caused by external or internal bleeding.
- Obstructive – e.g. tension pneumothorax, cardiac tamponade.
- Cardiogenic – resulting from blunt cardiac injury or myocardial infarction.
- Distributive – neurogenic or septic shock.

Of these, haemorrhagic shock requires the most urgent control.

The Lethal Triad (and Diamond)

Haemorrhage initiates a vicious cycle.

- Hypothermia caused by exposure and transfusion of cold fluids.
- Acidosis caused by inadequate perfusion.
- Coagulopathy caused by consumption of clotting factors and dilution from crystalloids.

This 'lethal triad' quickly worsens bleeding and raises the risk of death. Many now describe a 'lethal diamond', adding hypocalcaemia from massive transfusion as a fourth key factor.

Damage Control Resuscitation (DCR)

Modern trauma management emphasises DCR, which combines swift haemorrhage control with balanced transfusion and physiological optimisation.

Key principles include

- Permissive hypotension: in patients without TBI, aim for a systolic BP of 80–90 mmHg until haemorrhage is controlled, to prevent dislodging fragile clots. In patients with suspected TBI, maintain systolic BP ≥ 110 mmHg to ensure adequate cerebral perfusion.
- Haemostatic resuscitation: replace lost blood with balanced transfusion (packed red cells, plasma, platelets in a 1:1:1 ratio). Cryoprecipitate should be administered promptly if fibrinogen levels are low.
- Tranexamic acid (TXA): administer 1 g IV as soon as possible, followed by 1 g over 8 hours, ideally within 3 hours of injury, as recommended by the CRASH-2 trial and NICE guidance.
- Minimise crystalloids: large volumes of saline or Hartmann's worsen dilutional coagulopathy and acidosis.

Massive Transfusion Protocols

A massive transfusion protocol (MTP) should be activated early for patients presenting with life-threatening haemorrhage. These protocols facilitate rapid delivery of blood products to the bedside, enhance communication between clinical teams and the blood bank, and standardise transfusion ratios.

Indicators for activation may include

- Systolic BP <90 mmHg with evidence of ongoing bleeding.
- Positive FAST in the presence of haemodynamic instability.
- Transfusion of more than 4 units of red cells within the first hour.

Haemorrhage Control

While resuscitation continues, all efforts should be made to attain definitive haemorrhage control.

- External bleeding: tourniquets, haemostatic dressings, and direct pressure.
- Pelvic fractures: apply a pelvic binder at the level of the greater trochanters to reduce pelvic volume and tamponade bleeding. Early interventional radiology (embolisation) or surgical fixation may be necessary.
- Thoracic bleeding: use chest drains or perform emergency thoracotomy for massive haemothorax or cardiac tamponade.
- Abdominal bleeding: emergency laparotomy for splenic or hepatic injury not controlled by interventional radiology.
- Extremity bleeding: prompt involvement of orthopaedic or vascular surgery.

Adjunctive Monitoring

- Point-of-care coagulation testing (e.g. thromboelastography, ROTEM) guides transfusion more accurately than traditional clotting profiles.
- Serial blood gases enable monitoring of lactate and base deficit as indicators of perfusion.

The Role of Interventional Radiology

Advances in trauma care increasingly utilise interventional radiology for haemorrhage control. Embolisation of bleeding vessels, especially in pelvic and solid organ injuries, provides a minimally invasive alternative to open surgery, reducing morbidity and transfusion needs.

Special Trauma Considerations

Traumatic Brain Injury (TBI)

TBI is a major cause of death and disability after trauma. Even minor injuries can have long-lasting effects, whereas severe TBI demands immediate treatment to prevent secondary brain damage.

- Assessment: the GCS remains essential. Pupillary asymmetry or deterioration is very worrying.
- Management: maintain the airway and oxygenation, ensure normocapnia, and avoid hypotension (systolic BP less than 110 mmHg worsens outcomes). Hypertonic saline or mannitol may be used acutely if raised intracranial pressure (ICP) is suspected. Early CT and referral to neurosurgery are essential.
- Critical care: many patients need sedation, ventilation, and invasive ICP monitoring.

Chest Trauma

Thoracic injuries occur in 25% of serious trauma cases and directly cause up to a third of deaths. Early recognition of life-threatening conditions is essential.

- Tension pneumothorax and massive haemothorax necessitate immediate intervention (needle decompression and chest drains).
- Suspect cardiac tamponade in penetrating chest trauma presenting with shock and muffled heart sounds; while pericardiocentesis can be life-saving, thoracotomy remains the definitive treatment.
- Flail chest impairs ventilation and frequently necessitates intubation and analgesia.

Abdominal and Pelvic Trauma

Abdominal and pelvic injuries are significant causes of concealed haemorrhage.

- Abdominal trauma: FAST scanning or CT may detect solid organ injury (liver, spleen). Stable patients can be managed conservatively with observation and embolisation, whereas unstable patients often require laparotomy.
- Pelvic trauma: highly vascular and a common cause of exsanguination. Pelvic binders should be applied early, and interventional radiology or preperitoneal packing should be used where available.

Spinal Injuries

Spinal cord injury can occur in isolation or with polytrauma.

- Recognition: neurological assessment includes motor, sensory, and reflex functions. Neurogenic shock (hypotension and bradycardia) may mimic hypovolaemia but requires vasopressors rather than fluid overload.
- Management: spinal immobilisation until injury is excluded radiologically. Early spinal surgical consultation is essential.

Burns (Brief Overview)

Though less common in polytrauma, burns may complicate resuscitation.

- Airway: always consider inhalation injury in cases of facial burns or smoke inhalation.
- Circulation: fluid resuscitation guided by the Parkland formula, but avoid over-resuscitation ('fluid creep').
- Critical care: infection prevention and pain management are essential in long-term care.

Bibliography

Advanced Trauma Life Support (ATLS®). Student Course Manual. 10th ed. American College of Surgeons; 2018.

Bouillon B, Maegele M. Trauma care in Europe. Eur J Trauma Emerg Surg. 2019;45(6):815–826.

Brohi K, Singh J, Heron M, Coats T. Acute traumatic coagulopathy. J Trauma. 2003;54(6):1127–1130.

CRASH-2 Trial Collaborators. Effects of tranexamic acid on death, vascular occlusive events, and blood transfusion in trauma patients with significant haemorrhage (CRASH-2): a randomised, placebo-controlled trial. Lancet. 2010;376(9734):23–32.

European Society of Anaesthesiology and Intensive Care (ESAIC) & European Society of Intensive Care Medicine (ESICM). European Guideline on Management of Major Bleeding and Coagulopathy Following Trauma. Vol 27. 6th ed. Critical Care; 2023, p. 194.

National Institute for Health and Care Excellence (NICE). Major Trauma: Assessment and Initial Management. NICE Guideline [NG39]. London: NICE; 2016 (updated 2023).

Resuscitation Council UK. Trauma and Peri-arrest Algorithms. London: RCUK; 2021.

Royal College of Emergency Medicine (RCEM). Major Trauma Clinical Guidance. RCEM; 2022.

Vulliamy P, Brohi K. Damage control resuscitation. Br J Anaesth. 2017;119(1):i26–i34.

70

Ventilation

Mechanical ventilation supports patients who cannot breathe or oxygenate properly on their own. It is indicated in cases of respiratory failure, decreased consciousness, airway protection, or during anaesthesia for surgery. Ventilation can be invasive, using an endotracheal or tracheostomy tube, or non-invasive with snug-fitting masks. The primary objectives are to ensure effective gas exchange, reduce the effort of breathing, and allow time for recovery from the cause of respiratory failure.

Modes of Mechanical Ventilation

The choice of ventilatory mode relies on the patient's respiratory effort, underlying condition, and treatment objectives.

- Assist-control (AC): delivers a fixed number of fully supported breaths per minute. If the patient initiates a breath, the ventilator provides complete assistance. Offers full support but risks alkalosis if the patient hyperventilates.
- Synchronised intermittent mandatory ventilation (SIMV): provides mandatory breaths while permitting spontaneous unassisted (or pressure-supported) breaths between them. Useful during weaning.
- Pressure support ventilation (PSV): delivers a set pressure to assist each spontaneous breath. Commonly utilised during spontaneous breathing trials prior to extubation.
- Non-invasive modes
  - CPAP: continuous pressure maintained throughout the cycle, used in sleep apnoea and pulmonary oedema.
  - BiPAP: two pressure levels (higher during inspiration, lower during expiration), useful in hypercapnic failure such as COPD exacerbations.
- Advanced modes: e.g. APRV (airway pressure release ventilation) for ARDS, providing sustained high pressures with periodic releases while allowing spontaneous breathing.

Ventilator Settings Explained

- Tidal volume (V_t): typically, 6–8 mL/kg of ideal body weight; reduced to about 6 mL/kg in ARDS to minimise lung injury.
- Respiratory rate (RR): corrected for CO_2 removal.
- FiO_2: adjust to sustain sufficient oxygenation at the lowest safe concentration.

- PEEP: prevents alveolar collapse; baseline 5 cmH_2O, increased in severe hypoxaemia.
- I:E ratio: usually 1:2; longer expiratory times in obstructive disease to prevent air trapping.
- Pressures: maintain plateau pressure below 30 cmH_2O to minimise barotrauma. An increasing peak pressure, but a normal plateau, indicates airway resistance; if both are elevated, it suggests reduced compliance.

Clinical Considerations and Weaning

- ARDS: use lung-protective ventilation (low tidal volume, permissive hypercapnia, higher PEEP).
- COPD/asthma: encourage prolonged expiration to prevent dynamic hyperinflation.
- Neuromuscular weakness: offer full support at first, then switch to spontaneous modes as strength increases.
- Weaning: gradual decrease of support. Spontaneous breathing trials (PSV or T-piece) evaluate readiness, while monitoring for fatigue, poor gas exchange, or obstruction.

Risks and Monitoring

Although lifesaving, ventilation can pose potential risks.

- Infective: ventilator-associated pneumonia.
- Mechanical: barotrauma, volutrauma, or diaphragm atrophy.
- Haemodynamic: decreased venous return and hypotension, especially with high PEEP.

Regular assessment of ventilator settings, gas exchange, and patient comfort is vital. Decisions regarding initiation, escalation, or withdrawal of ventilation should always be made within a multidisciplinary team and aligned with the patient's overall care goals.

Bibliography

British Thoracic Society/Intensive Care Society. Guidelines for the ventilatory management of acute hypercapnic respiratory failure in adults. Thorax, Suppl 2. 2016;71:ii1–ii35.

Fan E, Beitler JR, Brochard L, et al. Lung protective ventilation in acute respiratory distress syndrome. JAMA. 2018;319(7):698–710.

Griffiths MJD, McAuley DF, Perkins GD, et al. Guidelines on the management of acute respiratory distress syndrome. BMJ Open Respir Res. 2019;6:e000420.

Marini JJ, Gattinoni L. Management of COVID-19 respiratory distress. JAMA. 2020;323(22):2329–2330.

NHS England. Guidance for the Provision of Mechanical Ventilation in Critical Care. NHS England; 2021.

NICE. Chronic Obstructive Pulmonary Disease in Over 16s: Diagnosis and Management. NICE Guideline [NG115]; 2019.

Slutsky AS, Ranieri VM. Ventilator-induced lung injury. N Engl J Med. 2013;369(22):2126–2136.

71

Well-Being and Resilience in Healthcare Professionals

Healthcare is a rewarding profession, but it also poses physical, emotional, and psychological demands. Long hours, high-stakes decision-making, and exposure to suffering and death can impact staff at all levels. Well-being is not merely a personal issue but a professional and organisational priority, as it directly affects patient care, safety, and workforce sustainability. Resilience, the ability to adapt and recover when faced with challenges, is increasingly recognised as an essential trait for clinicians. This chapter discusses the significance of well-being, the challenges encountered, and strategies for developing resilience within healthcare practice.

The Pressures of Healthcare

Modern healthcare environments are fast-paced and often under-resourced. Staff shortages, increasing patient demand, and administrative burdens can lead to chronic stress. In acute and emergency care settings, the intensity is heightened by time-critical decisions, unpredictable workloads, and exposure to traumatic events. Emotional strain is worsened by moral dilemmas, such as balancing limited resources or making end-of-life decisions. If these pressures are not addressed, they can result in burnout, fatigue, compassion fatigue, and ultimately staff leaving the profession.

Burnout and Its Consequences

Burnout is characterised by emotional exhaustion, depersonalisation, and a reduced sense of personal achievement. It is linked to anxiety, depression, and physical ill health, but its impact also reaches patient outcomes. Clinicians experiencing burnout are more prone to make errors, have diminished empathy, and deliver lower-quality care. Recognising burnout early and addressing its causes is therefore essential for both personal well-being and patient safety.

Building Resilience

Resilience does not mean being unaffected by stress or adversity; rather, it reflects the ability to recover and continue functioning effectively in the face of stress or adversity. It can be developed at both an individual and organisational level. On a personal level, maintaining healthy lifestyle habits-adequate sleep, regular exercise, and balanced nutrition-supports both physical and mental well-being. Building strong support networks among colleagues, friends, and family provides a buffer against stress. Reflective practice, mindfulness, and stress management techniques can also enhance coping capacity.

At an organisational level, resilience is fostered by creating supportive environments where staff feel valued and safe to speak out. Providing access to debriefing after challenging cases, offering counselling services, and encouraging flexible working patterns all help staff manage their roles' demands. Leadership plays a vital role in modelling healthy behaviours, reducing stigma around mental health, and ensuring that well-being is integrated into workplace culture.

Work–Life Balance

Maintaining a sustainable balance between professional responsibilities and personal life is vital for well-being. The unpredictable hours and shift work common in healthcare can disrupt relationships, social activities, and rest. Protecting time outside of work for relaxation and personal fulfilment helps prevent professional stress from taking over all aspects of life. While achieving a perfect balance may not always be feasible, recognising the importance of time away from work and setting boundaries where possible can help reduce the risk of chronic fatigue and burnout.

Moral Injury and Compassion Fatigue

Alongside burnout, healthcare workers may experience moral injury – the distress that arises when clinicians feel unable to act in accordance with their ethical or professional values, such as when resource limitations prevent the delivery of optimal care. Similarly, compassion fatigue may occur when repeated exposure to suffering reduces a clinician's capacity for empathy. Both can undermine professional identity and personal well-being. Addressing these issues requires organisational recognition, open discussion, and strategies to support staff in processing these experiences.

Strategies for Supporting Well-Being

A variety of strategies can encourage and safeguard the well-being of healthcare professionals.

- Education and training: integrating well-being and resilience training into medical and nursing curricula helps normalise these discussions and arms staff with tools from the beginning of their careers.

- Peer support and mentoring: formal mentorship schemes and informal peer support can help staff feel less isolated and more connected.
- Access to psychological support: confidential counselling and occupational health services should be readily available without stigma.
- Reflective practice: regular opportunities to reflect – individually or in groups – encourage processing of experiences and continual growth.
- Organisational culture: institutions that prioritise well-being by addressing workload, valuing staff, and promoting inclusivity foster a healthier workforce.

Well-being and resilience are not optional extras for healthcare professionals; they are crucial for providing safe, effective, and compassionate care. While individuals can take steps to enhance their resilience, organisations also bear the responsibility to create environments where staff are supported, valued, and able to flourish. By prioritising well-being, the healthcare sector can maintain not only the health of its workforce but also the quality of care given to patients.

Bibliography

General Medical Council (GMC). Caring for Doctors, Caring for Patients. London: GMC; 2019.

Maslach C, Leiter MP. Understanding the burnout experience: recent research and its implications for psychiatry. World Psych. 2016;15(2):103–111.

Royal College of Nursing (RCN). Staff Wellbeing and Resilience. London: RCN; 2022.

Shanafelt TD, Noseworthy JH. Executive leadership and physician well-being: nine organisational strategies to promote engagement and reduce burnout. Mayo Clin Proc. 2017;92(1):129–146.

West M, Coia D. Caring for Doctors, Caring for Patients: How to Transform UK Healthcare Environments to Support Doctors and Medical Students to Thrive. London: GMC; 2019.

Index

i

q

r

www.ingramcontent.com/pod-product-compliance
Lightning Source LLC
LaVergne TN
LVHW080846170826
845678LV00006B/1726

* 9 7 8 1 3 9 4 3 0 3 9 3 9 *